Lunar Abundance

Reflective Journal

Lunar Abundance

Reflective Journal

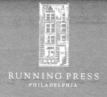

YOUR GUIDEBOOK TO WORKING WITH THE PHASES OF THE MOON

EZZIE SPENCER, PhD

RUNNING PRESS

PHILADELPHIA

Running Press
Hachette Book Group
1290 Avenue of the Americas, New York, NY 10104
www.runningpress.com
@Running_Press

Printed in China

First Edition: December 2019

Published by Running Press, an imprint of Perseus Books, LLC, a subsidiary of Hachette Book Group, Inc. The Running Press name and logo is a trademark of the Hachette Book Group.

The Hachette Speakers Bureau provides a wide range of authors for speaking events. To find out more, go to www.hachettespeakersbureau.com or call (866) 376-6591.

The publisher is not responsible for websites (or their content) that are not owned by the publisher.

Photographs by Emma-Kate Codrington

Library of Congress Control Number: 2019943999

ISBNs: 978-0-7624-6850-8

RRD-S

10 9 8 7 6 5 4 3 2 1

For all the
Lunar Abundance
moon-gazers around
the world.

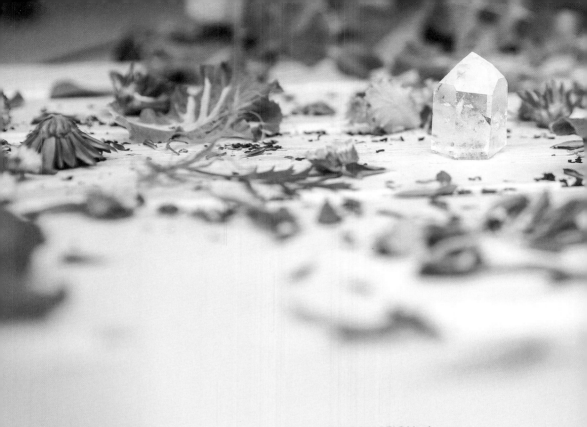

Contents

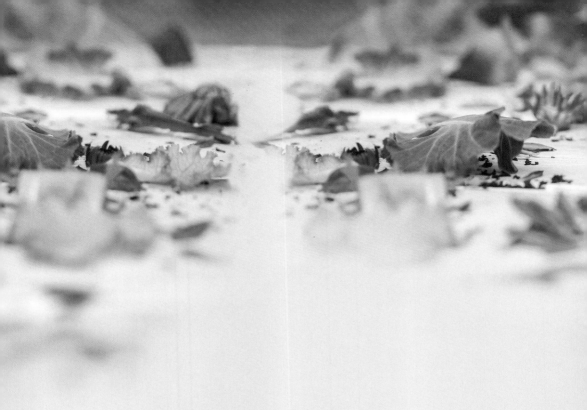

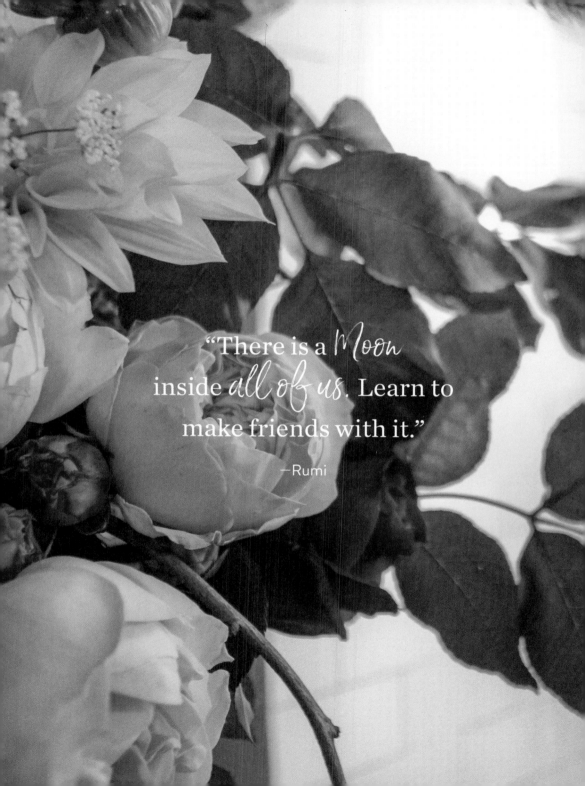

"There is a *Moon* inside *all of us*. Learn to make friends with it."

—Rumi

INTRODUCTION

Since ancient times, we have sensed the magic of the Moon. (We are cyclical creatures, after all.)

But it is only when you begin harnessing the power of the Moon cycle to create a life of abundance that you truly discover the Moon-magic that exists *within you*. As the Moon reflects light from the Sun, it also illuminates your soul's hidden wisdom.

When people practice Lunar Abundance, there are typically two types of results. The first is that you may start to effortlessly draw toward you tangible things like more money, clients, new soul friends, a new home, a soul mate or intimate partner, greater health and well-being, a new job, a pregnancy—or whatever you set as your New Moon intention each month. The second type of benefit is also welcome. You will start to become calmer and more peaceful, more relaxed, more joyful, and more attuned to your soul purpose. You will start to uncover the keys to working with less effort, and live with ease and flow. You may find that you cultivate qualities like kindness, compassion, love, and forgiveness, which means that you have a positive ripple effect in your family, workplace, and others in your orbit.

This practice has transformed my own life. It has meant that I've gone from being a stressed-out lawyer, sitting in an office in Sydney, Australia, to traveling the world, supporting myself through meaningful work, prioritizing self-care, and connecting with my global soul family.

While I have carefully designed key elements of my life, it is actually even better than I could have imagined because this practice also creates space for . . . magic. My younger self would have laughed if someone had told me I would be working in New York City—as a modern "Moon Goddess," among other things—in my thirties.

My secret? I didn't look out; I looked in. I followed the crumbs to my dreams using a specific process, as you will be guided to do yourself through the pages of this journal.

So how does it work? What is the link between the Moon and abundance? Well, the Moon represents our subconscious. Most of us, however, have only been taught how to create abundance through conscious means. We work hard, do all the right things, but often don't feel ourselves experiencing results in the way we would like.

Why? Well, oftentimes our subconscious is driving our behavior more than we realize.

While many are attracted to lunar principles because we want to live in a natural state of flow, when it comes to creating our dreams, we still tend to cling to pushing, hustling, and striving, often burning ourselves out in the process.

With Lunar Abundance, we bring the subconscious mind into play. Many love how simple, yet profound, the practice is. Rather than just thinking about what you want and doing some things you think will help you achieve your intention, Lunar Abundance teaches you how to harness the potency of your feelings to attract and hold more abundance in your life.

The result? Creating abundance becomes a much easier—not to mention more joyful—process.

Whatever your relationship to the Moon right now; whether you barely notice her waxing and waning above, or you observe her cycles religiously, by using this guidebook, you will discover the depth of your power.

It's important to acknowledge that the entire breadth and depth of Lunar Abundance is not taught within these pages. Rather, this journal guides your reflections as you follow the eight phases of the Moon. You will find many more examples, case studies, resources, and the depths of the practice contained in my first book, *Lunar Abundance* (Running Press, 2018).

This journal is a tool for self-inquiry, so please know that wherever you are right now is perfect. If you are already working with the Lunar Abundance practice, this book will enrich your experience. And if you are new to the principles of Lunar Abundance, this is a wonderful tool to start putting some basic principles into practice.

Please remember: You are not striving to achieve. As you follow the advice and journal prompts for each of the eight Moon phases, bear in mind that Lunar Abundance is not about becoming a "better person." Self-improvement is not the goal. Understanding your soul purpose is. Once we tune in to our own feelings, we create an internal foundation for calling in and holding on to the opportunities that are truly aligned with who we really are.

At the New Moon each month, I hold a ceremony either online or in the city where I reside (at the moment, New York City). I've been holding these events for nearly a decade. This means that I have now led tens of thousands of people around the world into the Lunar Abundance practice.

Over time, I have become more attuned to what readers need to know about how to use this practice (which I originally created for myself) to make magic in *your own* life.

The purpose of the *Lunar Abundance Reflective Journal* is to help you to implement the teachings and learnings from the Lunar Abundance practice in a simple and practical, everyday way, to guide you in seeing your own dreams come true.

WHY PRACTICE LUNAR ABUNDANCE?

●

●

◖

◖

You might be curious about the Moon cycle. As a little girl, I was *fascinated* by it. When I started working consciously with the Moon's cycle, I was delighted to discover that I could do more than simply gaze at it in the night sky and admire its beauty. It held more. When I aligned with the Moon cycle, it held a kind of mystical power for me.

I found the Moon to be a mirror that reflected my own power. The Lunar Abundance practice is ultimately a way for us to chart our own course in life. It is not about the Moon *making* us do anything! It's about coming within and accessing our own intuition, wisdom, and personal power. You might feel that there is a secret life that you could be leading—your true life. One with a greater sense of purpose. One that feels authentically yours.

Do you ask yourself: Why am I really here on Earth? What am I here to do? Am I living the life I really want to lead? And how might I go about creating that dream life for myself, and others in my orbit?

This book provides a simple guide for this journey. The first chapter, the New Moon, will invite you to dare to dream about something bigger. It will inspire your imagination so you can start dreaming about *what* you want to create in your life, and gain clarity on *why* you want to create it. The following chapters

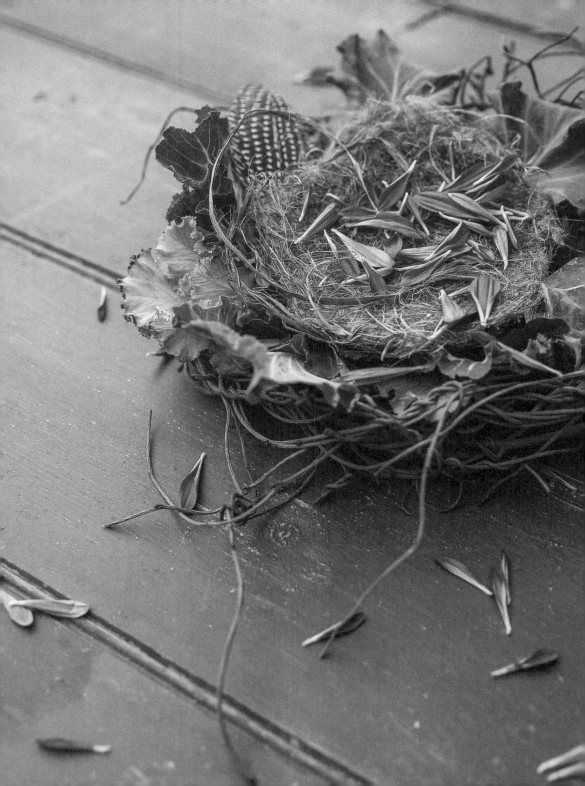

then show you *how* to create that life by giving you practical tools and exercises to start making real change.

The best part is that the Lunar Abundance practice offers a more sustainable path to success than simply going through the motions. The increasing demands of modern life may leave you stressed and anxious. You may be overwhelmed with more and more demands on your attention. You may feel as if you're struggling, and you may be wishing for greater ease. You may have an urgent need to calm down to get through the day and work effectively, or you may feel a deeper yearning for an inner state of peace and harmony. You may wish for things to be easier. I know that I did.

If you were anything like me, you also may feel a sense that there is something *more* out there. You may feel a sense of loneliness and disconnection from others. You may feel disconnected from nature. Ultimately, you may feel disconnected from yourself—and from the joy that is your birthright.

My Story

Before we start, let me tell you how Lunar Abundance came to be. I spent my twenties walking the line of burnout. Drinking, partying, and working myself into the ground were all big distractions for me so I didn't have to face what was going on inside me.

Sure, my work was meaningful, but I was run by stress and anxiety, and partly motivated by achievement. This was at the expense of my health, both physical and emotional. It was at the expense of my happiness. My power. My true purpose.

As a kind of personal therapy, I spontaneously started to track the Moon in my mid-twenties. The lunar cycle became my anchor, a guide. I would just look up at night, see which phase it was in, check the sign, write about how I was feeling, and note correlations with my life. Over time, I recognized patterns in my mood, my own emotional tides.

I found lunar tracking to be a safe and gentle way to come back into connection with myself.

I found peace and understanding through tracking the Moon—and started to come into a more meaningful and loving relationship with myself and my body's wisdom.

This is because the Moon represents the *feelings*.

But then there was more.

The Moon also represents the *subconscious*, and once I had lunar tracking down, I started to play with the Moon in deeper and more creative ways that tapped into this. By following certain principles—setting intentions, leaning back, taking discerning action, trusting, letting go, expressing gratitude, giving back, and reflecting—I started to connect more deeply with abundance principles. The Moon cycle became my timekeeper, my guide.

I began to align with the lunar cycle to do the inner work that is necessary to cultivate a true state of abundance. I started to speak about what I was becoming. It became a coaching business when people started to ask how they could work with me to learn these principles, too, and my life started to shift quite dramatically.

Lunar Abundance evolved from researching, experimenting, implementing, and reflecting. Then repeating, teaching, and learning some more. I developed it because I had to find a way to escape the chronic stress and overwhelm I experienced when working in my first career. At key points in designing this practice, my creation was influenced in various ways by Steven Forrest, Megan Davis, Kevin Farrow, Sandra Mosley, Saida Desilets, and Tom Starke.

There are many ways to follow the Moon. Lunar Abundance is my personal practice. I developed it because I had to find a way to escape the chronic stress and overwhelm when working in my first career. I tell the detailed story of how

I discovered certain elements in my original book on Lunar Abundance.

My tens of thousands of readers and clients have been generous teachers for me over the years. And my intuition, my feelings, have been my guide. Always, I've been influenced by Lady Luna.

Getting the Most from Lunar Abundance

One of the things that I love about Lunar Abundance is that it is so simple, and yet profound. It is extremely powerful—if you do the inner work (the basics of which are shared in this journal).

Lunar Abundance is based on the Hermetic principle of correspondence: as above, so below. This means that the Moon reflects your own emotions and feelings. I don't believe that the Moon *makes* you do or feel anything. It is simply a mirror that helps you notice what's already going on inside.

Unfurling this Lunar Abundance practice involves deep self-love, honest self-inquiry, action, and reflection.

This practice helps you to connect with your soul. It helps you deepen your intuition and self-knowing. It guides you into meaningful and fruitful dialogue with your subconscious. And if you do the work, it will allow the energy of abundance to flow more smoothly. When I talk about abundance, I am not just using this word as another word for "money." I mean a way of being (with certain thoughts, and actions, flowing from this in turn). The word "abundance" itself comes from the Latin word meaning "overflow." One of the core characteristics of abundance is being in the flow. Clients and readers routinely share that the Lunar Abundance practice has helped them to ride the surging waves of life, to embody the understanding that abundance is about receiving energy and joy and love, and that it's also about sharing the good vibes of this overflow with others.

Most of all, abundance involves a deep knowing that everything *is okay*. Living in abundance means that you fully internalize this knowing—not that it *will be* okay, but that it *is* okay.

To see results, you need to do the inner work. You can do this with guidance, and with support, but it's mostly up to you. You need to be devoted to the practice, but, I assure you, it is a very simple, gentle, low-maintenance one that is easy to incorporate in your life.

Follow all the steps at each of the eight phases throughout each lunar cycle.

Your intuition and capacity to *be* is like a muscle. You may start to see the positive effects of the practice, but if you veer away from it for too long, your newfound magical powers will start to subside. Then it's time to return to the practice. Lunar Abundance is both preparation for and goes hand-in-hand with a deep soul journey.

I intentionally developed Lunar Abundance as an easy, feel-good, and gentle practice. My life at the time was such a grind that I knew I needed to develop a beautiful practice for myself that would not take a huge amount of time and effort and that I felt *inspired* to follow each day.

This journal has been intentionally designed not to overwhelm you with excessive information. It's necessary for me to set out the key principles in the New Moon chapter to frame the practice, but Lunar Abundance is not something that you do with your mind. When you are seeking joy, peace, and purpose, your mind alone won't get you there. Your mind is a gateway to something far more magical, and it has brought you here, to this experience.

Lunar Abundance truly is something that you *experience*. The results will come from you showing up, by following this magical practice, and by writing out your answers to the prompts, rather than just reading them and thinking about them in your head. I have observed that those who record their observations and then reflect on them are the ones who see the best results. That's why I felt there was a need for this companion journal to my original book. Share your reflections with like-minded people. Be witnessed, be held accountable, and be supported.

This is not a one-lunar-cycle-and-you've-got-it kind of practice. No need to rush, and definitely do not push. Allow yourself to blossom, and unfurl, at the right pace for you. Lunar Abundance is a cumulative practice.

Each lunar cycle starts at the New Moon and lasts for about a month, comprising eight phases. Each lunar phase lasts three to four days, depending on the Moon's elliptical orbit, and these phases are observable and trackable throughout the lunar cycle. Just go outside at night and look up, or download the free lunar planner from my website, LunarAbundance.com.

At the New Moon, you set your intention. Sit with your intention for just one minute in meditation, each day. And then follow the steps that will come at each of the succeeding seven lunar phases. There are phases for *Being*, and phases for *Doing*. The original Lunar Abundance book provides the deep dive into the Being and Doing phases. In brief here:

Being: times to draw back, to reflect, to integrate, to process

Doing: times to move forward, to take action, to give

These phases are guides. Over time, you will find that these times can guide your schedule.

And, as you will discover, each of these phases is relative. It can take a while to fully align with the Moon cycle, but I invite you to actually do the work, and follow the steps. If you lose track, no need to worry. Be kind to yourself. Life happens! But don't use busyness as an excuse to abandon the practice. If you're reading this, it's because you want this.

What you will learn about yourself—what you will learn about your soul purpose—during the Lunar Abundance process is key to deeper soul development. It is about the means, not solely the ends. It is as much about the journey as it is about the destination.

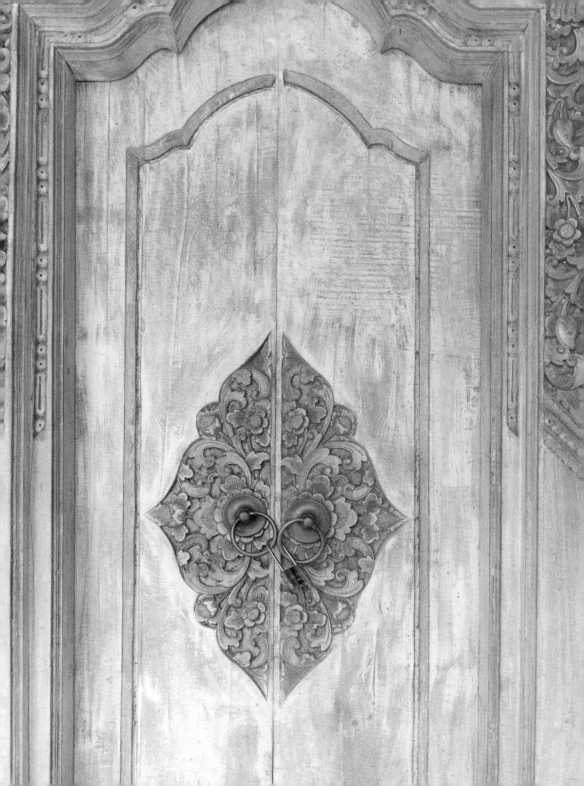

Each New Moon

Set a thematic, positive, feeling-based
intention for that lunar cycle.

Make it just about you.

☾

Create a Life of Abundance

Create a life of abundance by doing certain
things at *doing* lunar phases; and being a certain
way at *being* lunar phases.

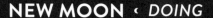

NEW MOON ‹ *DOING*

I set my intention. I feel my intention in my body.

CRESCENT MOON ‹ *BEING*

I relax into my intention. I breathe.

FIRST QUARTER MOON ‹ *DOING*

I take discerning action to support my intention.

GIBBOUS MOON ‹ *BEING*

I trust that the perfect intention is coming into form at the perfect time.

FULL MOON ‹ *DOING*

I move ahead with my intention now, OR I accept that my intention was not for the best at this time. I release it, and course-correct now.

DISSEMINATING MOON ‹ *BEING*

I feel grateful that my intention is coming into form in the perfect way. I receive with gratitude.

THIRD QUARTER MOON ‹ *DOING*

Now that I am receiving my intention, I give back from a place of abundance.

BALSAMIC MOON ‹ *BEING*

I reflect with thanks. I rest. I restore.

"My life didn't please me, so I created my life."

—*Coco Chanel*

New Moon

☾

"I set my intention. I feel my intention in my body."

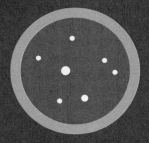

Even before the first sliver of moonlight is visible in the sky, the night energy feels potent and palpable. The reason we set intentions at the New Moon is because this is the start of the Moon cycle, and the start is the perfect time for setting authentic, delicious intentions. This chapter sets out the principles of intention-setting, and follows with journal prompts that will lead you through your own intention-setting process.

Intention-Setting Principles

You will start your practice by setting one very simple intention at the New Moon. You can easily work with a small and achievable intention over one Moon cycle, which is about a month, and see quick results.

I have found that when people set multiple intentions at the New Moon, it becomes overwhelming to follow the practice. And this practice is designed to help you find more simplicity and joy in life—not more stress! When you set multiple intentions, what usually happens is that it becomes "too hard," and you will abandon the practice.

For best results, set your New Moon intention in the special Lunar Abundance way, and then follow the steps laid out for you in this journal over the entire Moon cycle.

Can't decide which intention to choose? Well, the journaling prompts below will lead you through finding this. The simple answer, though, is to choose the intention that makes you feel *alive*.

Lunar Abundance intention-setting is feeling-based.

I invite you to set an intention that starts with the words "I feel . . ." This is because this practice is all about coming into an intimate relationship with your feelings. And by "feelings," I mean physical sensations in our body. The sensations are the pathway back into the body, into your subconscious mind, and into what you believe deep down. This practice shows you exactly how to rewrite any old inherited beliefs that aren't serving your growth and expansion in this life.

Feelings are different from emotions. What I mean by "emotions" is the meaning and interpretation you give to these sensations.

Rather than be at the whim of your emotions and at the mercy of your mood, this New Moon intention-setting process provides you with an opportunity to practice stepping into the power position with respect to your own emotional well-being. The easiest way I have found to step into your personal power is to anchor your intention in your body, by linking your New Moon intention to physical sensations and elevated emotions.

This is why I recommend that you link your intention to an emotion that makes you feel *great*—because your New Moon intention becomes an opportunity to practice sitting behind your own emotional dashboard and turning the right dials before your journey starts. You will save so much time and energy on your journey by ensuring that you know where you are going and that everything is correctly set before you start on your journey.

The purpose of linking your intention to an elevated emotion is not simply to feel good, it is so that you *most effectively* point yourself in the new direction that you want to go. This is because the best New Moon intentions come from the yearnings of your heart. Dreams do not exist in reality yet. However, when you use your subconscious to trick your conscious mind into thinking that your intention is already true, then you will start to feel in your body what it would be like to actually live the reality that you are creating for yourself.

Throughout the Moon cycle, your New Moon intention will be your compass. Tuning into it will help you recognize the right opportunities, which means you can use your intention as the compass to make the right decisions, and take effective action to make your dreams come true.

If you *feel* that your intention has already come true, you will start to build cellular memory related to your intention. When you have cellular memory, it just becomes second nature.

Personally, I have found that the single most powerful elevated emotion is gratitude. Carrying that into an example, your New Moon intention might be framed like this:

"I feel grateful as I receive . . . [fill in the blank]."

This is just one idea—one set of possible words—for framing your intention. Feel free to improvise. Other ideas include substituting "joy," "merriment," "happiness," and "laughter," in place of "grateful."

Play around with what works for you! Just remember to keep it simple, and make sure that it really does make you feel alive, and is *positive*.

Daniel Wegner, PhD, a psychology professor at Harvard University, once conducted an experiment in which the researchers asked participants *not* to think about a white bear. So what happened? All they could think about was white bears. Similarly, if you focus on letting go of fear (or anger, resentment, etc.) at the New Moon, you'll keep anchoring to—and therefore expanding feelings of—fear (or anger, resentment, etc.).

On the other hand, if you focus on welcoming in joy, gratitude, and love, you'll keep anchoring into—and therefore expanding feelings of—joy, happiness, and love, all month long.

Which would you prefer?

This *anchoring* will become more important throughout the Moon cycle, as you will see. Importantly, this approach is not the same as denying or bypassing our "negative" emotions. Keep in mind that I have designed Lunar Abundance like this for specific reasons.

Imagine that your current desire is to start a new business and you're really scared about that. Don't suppress your fear. *Note it.* Your honesty and self-awareness are extremely helpful at this stage because they direct you right toward a solution.

Your fear will help you craft an effective intention.
Remember: The cure is in the problem.

What is the opposite of fear? Or, what might help you navigate fear? Rather than setting a New Moon intention like this:

"I release fear about starting my new business!"

Try this:

"My shoulders move back and I feel grateful for my increasing ability to tap into my internal reservoir of courage as a successful business owner."

Or:

"I feel deep confidence fire up in my belly as I welcome a successful new business."

See the difference?

Can you see how we linked together our desired dream or outcome (to start a new, successful business), anchored it in physical sensations in specific parts of our body (referencing how we feel in the shoulders and belly), linked this with *elevated emotions* (gratitude and joy), and found *cures* (courage and confidence) inside the problem itself (fear)?

The reason fear is a problem here is that it will either block your success in bringing your intention to fruition, or it will block your ease and enjoyment in the process because it will feel like pushing a rock uphill. A block is linked to a belief that lives in our subconscious mind, where we can't easily find it, and it makes our life and work feel like a struggle.

In fact, many of us are addicted to struggle. But it doesn't have to be that way.

In Lunar Abundance, we do not use our conscious mind to go down the rabbit hole to find and analyze beliefs. We use a faster, more effective strategy to simply notice what we are feeling (in this case, fear), accept that this fear will block our progress (or our ease and enjoyment), thank the fear for pointing us in the direction of the cure, and then use our New Moon intention-setting process to dissolve the block and change the belief. We then start to make our dreams come true, with less effort, by drawing our dreams to us in a joyful, sustainable way.

These are some of the reasons that the Lunar Abundance practice feels good *and* brings results in the external world. Put simply, when you set a New Moon intention in the way that I explain, linking your desired outcome to an elevated emotion, and anchoring it to physical sensations in your body, you are onto a winning intention-setting formula.

The final thing to remember before you set a New Moon intention is to make it all about you.

This is for two reasons. First, we don't want to interfere with the free will of others, *even* if we think we are helping them. This practice is powerful, and I have coded it so it cannot be used to affect anyone else without their permission. Not only will your New Moon intention fail if you try to manipulate anyone (or even subtly "help" them), but it will also *feel bad* for you. Secondly, Lunar Abundance is a self-knowledge and self-care practice, among other things. The more that you set your New Moon intentions, the more you will come into greater relationship with what *you* want and need. This will profoundly change your life, as you build self-sovereignty and you won't be able to be manipulated by others for *their* benefit.

This is a crucial life skill not taught in school, but it is essential in a rapidly changing world, with many people out for your energy, your money, and your attention for reasons that may not be in your best interest. This practice shows you how to protect yourself, not by erecting barriers out of fear, but by understanding who you really are, what you feel, and what you need and want. So, make your New Moon intention wholly about you.

You spend so much time in your life giving to others (we'll get to that later in the practice, too). Right now, this is your chance to connect with, and give to, *yourself.*

SUMMARY OF INTENTION-SETTING

1. Set one intention (that is, don't try to radically overhaul your entire life in one Moon cycle).
2. Link your intention to a feeling in your body (a physical sensation).
3. Link your intention to an elevated emotion (such as gratitude, savoring, or joy).
4. Write down your New Moon intention in the positive (welcome in, not release).
5. Make sure your New Moon intention is all about *you.*

We set our intentions at the New Moon because intentions are best to set at the start, and the New Moon is the start of the Moon cycle.

In Lunar Abundance, we set our intentions in a very specific way, for very specific reasons linked to the true meaning and gifts of this practice. I am about to lead you through the process step-by-step, from generating ideas to formulating a draft intention to unlocking your own personal, authentic, and beautiful New Moon intention.

You will receive extra guidance in this section, as I want to set you up for true success on your lunar journey. So get your pen out, relax, and get ready to flow into the magic!

JOURNAL PROMPTS FOR THE NEW MOON

When is the next New Moon? Download the free lunar planner from my website, LunarAbundance.com, and write down the date of the next New Moon here:

....

‹ Lunar Abundance is a cure for loneliness and disconnection. The practice fosters connection to natural rhythms and cycles, connection to others, and connection to yourself. Do you plan to set your New Moon intention by yourself, or will you invite together a group of people to do this together? It is perfectly fine to do it by yourself, and you may wish to do that in your first cycle. If you choose to invite others, who will you invite?

....

....

....

....

....

....

....

....

‹ At this perfect time for setting your intention, where will you choose to be? Where could you feel safe, relaxed, and receptive to internal wisdom? List all the possibilities.

....

....

....

....

....

....

....

....

....

‹   Which one location feels like the right choice for you at this upcoming New Moon phase? (This may change from cycle to cycle.) Specify that location here:

....

....

....

....

....

‹   A key principle of Lunar Abundance is to feel your intentions, rather than simply thinking about them. The act of feeling your intention charges it with power beyond mere thought. Sit now, close your eyes, and breathe deeply. Observe the physical sensations in your body. By tuning in to your feelings, direct your attention to the part of your body that feels warm and tingly.

Whether you feel it in your hips or your heart or somewhere else entirely, record that sensation, and its location.

....

....

....

....

....

....

....

....

....

....

....

‹   Now that you are anchored in your body, consider what you most desire. Is there something in your life that is *not* working, something you would like to change? Do you love your work? Are you happy where you live? Do you have an intimate relationship with someone you love? Do you have enough money in your bank account? Are you as creative as you desire?

If it feels as if there is something missing in your life, rather than feeling worried or despairing about it, you can see this feeling as a helpful clue to direct you toward what you want to welcome in. Write down all the areas of your life that you wish were different.

....

....

....

....

....

....

....

....

....

....

....

....

....

☾ Now consider *why* you want these things to be different. What is underpinning your desires? For example, is desiring money in your bank account really about needing security? Is wanting a partner really about needing to receive love and affection? Is wishing that you didn't detest your work really about needing to fulfill your soul purpose?

The invitation is to be curious here—not to think that you shouldn't want these things, but to be open and honest with yourself about what is truly underlying your desires.

What you write here will inform your authentic New Moon intention, so heartstorm here:

....

....

....

....

....

....

....

....

....

....

....

....

....

....

....

....

....

....
....
....
....
....
....
....
....
....
....
....
....

❮ Consider now what is really working beautifully in your life at this time. For example, are your friendships going great? Is your job meaningful and fulfilling? Are you making good money? Are you loving your home? What would you like to keep going, or want more of?

Take a moment to note what you would like to expand now. Record these observations here:

....
....
....
....
....
....
....
....
....
....

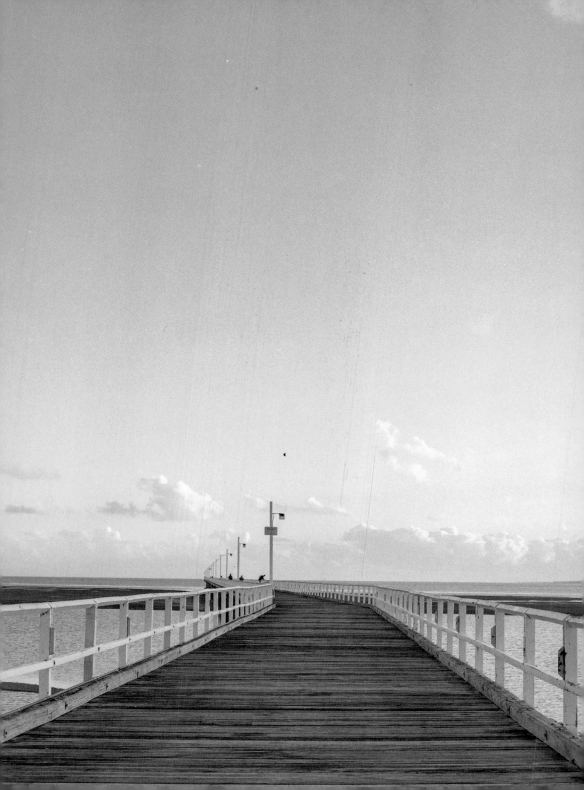

It is *intention-setting* time! Go *deep*, feel *within*, and set an *intention*.

‹ Consider now which of your needs are already met by the parts of your life that are working. For example, is your social circle or family meeting your need for love and connection? Does your home help you feel safe and grounded? Does your physical health help you feel vital and alive? Does your job help you feel that you are making a meaningful contribution to the world?

Write down everything you feel grateful for in your life, and your needs that are already met.

Now it's time to breathe deeply. We have intentionally stirred up many thoughts and feelings, which will be very useful as we weave into the New Moon intention-setting process.

If you would like more support with a guided process, you may wish to download the New Moon audio meditation from my website, LunarAbundance.com. Or you may wish to close your eyes, bow your head to your heart, and simply ask yourself:

"What is my New Moon intention for this Moon cycle?"

❮ Pause, feel deeply, and listen for the answer. Then return here. Write down everything that just came up for you (we will get clarity soon).

....

....

....

....

....

....

....

....

....

....

....

....

....

....

❬ Did your answers surprise you? Is there anything you felt that you haven't written down? Don't hold back. You don't need to censor yourself, and you definitely do not need to rush this process. Record here now what else came up for you this time.

....

....

....

....

....

....

....

....

....

....

❬ Next, review the list above. What one facet of your life did you write down that makes you feel most alive in your body? Record that here:

....

....

....

....

....

....

....

....

....

....

....

....

....

....

....

‹ What did you actually *feel* in your body when you chose that one intention? By that I mean, what physical sensations did you feel when you paid attention to what you wrote above? Describe these physical sensations in detail, and link them to specific body parts, such as your chest or your toes. We are practicing body awareness, which is how we will anchor our intention in our cells. Record your observations about your physical sensations.

....

....

....

....

....

....

....

....

....

....

....

....

....

❬ What were the emotions that came up for you during this intention-setting process? This invitation is to be curious and not judgmental. If you felt frustrated, write that down. If you felt sad or angry, write that down. You do not need to get upset for feeling what you feel, and you never need to censor yourself in this journal.

The more open and honest you are, the more easily you will alchemize these emotions. If you are feeling uncomfortable, please know that the next section offers a transformational pathway to any emotions that you wish to productively work through.

Be specific as possible when you name your emotions here now. And be kind to yourself!

....

....

....

....

....

....

....

....

....

....

....

....

....

....

....

....

Review your list of emotions. Does it include emotions that you can link back to physical sensations? The opportunity here is to name your emotions, rather than visualizations ("I felt golden" is an example of a thought or visualization, not an emotion).

I invite you to go deeper than the thought, and into the emotion itself. This is because when we use mental devices to avoid our feelings, we can miss out on the richness of what our feelings are trying to tell us. Lunar Abundance is designed to help us start to touch this deeper and powerful feeling dimension of ourselves—in a very safe and gentle way. For example, "golden" is a nice thought that might trigger an emotion of excitement, awe, glee, or happiness. So in this instance, you would write "excitement" rather than "golden."

If this is a challenge, that is a good thing! You are amplifying your emotional fluency!

☾ Review your list above and go deeper into any thoughts and into the emotions behind them now. Record them here:

....
....
....
....
....
....
....
....
....
....
....
....
....

....
....
....
....
....
....
....
....
....
....
....
....
....
....
....
....
....

Now consider the following: Are you feeling what you *want* to feel? If not, what might be the opposite of that emotion, or an emotion to support the emotion that you are currently feeling? For example, if you are feeling scared, how does it feel to set an intention to feel safe, or confident? If you are feeling lonely and isolated, what about feeling connection and joy? If you are feeling anxious, how might it feel to set an intention to feel peace and calm?

The cure is in the problem!

Please also know that if you are feeling sadness, there is nothing wrong with that. Many start to cry as we connect with our true selves, and tears can be so healing. Indeed, there is nothing wrong with feeling any "negative" emotion.

This is a transformational practice that will show you how to use your emotions as clues toward understanding yourself, and making any necessary changes.

‹ Even if you can't access any elevated emotions right now, take a moment to look at what you've written down above, and invert these emotions to discover what you *could* feel. Record it here:

....
....
....
....
....
....
....
....
....
....
....
....
....
....
....
....
....
....
....

◖ Next, write down the first draft of your New Moon intention here. You may wish to start with the words "I feel . . ."

....

....

....

....

....

....

....

....

....

....

....

....

....

Now review. Does your written intention include references to feelings (physical sensations)? If not, please take another moment to feel your intention in your body now. Can you feel specific physical sensations (such as tingling) in specific body parts? If you can't feel anything in your body at all, please know that this can also be a win! You may be noticing for the first time that you are numb. Be kind to yourself, if this is what you notice. Self-awareness is the first step in transformation. Without honesty and awareness, we can't change. This practice will then lead you through the next steps about *how* to change.

If you can't feel anything at all (or if you are only feeling painful sensations), then I invite you to brainstorm what pleasurable physical sensations you would *like* to feel. For example, you may wish to feel warmth in your heart and toes.

‹ Now I invite you to rewrite your New Moon intention here so that it makes reference to physical sensations. Or, set an intention to *feel* pleasurable physical sensations this cycle:

....

....

....

....

....

....

....

....

....

....

....

....

‹ If your written New Moon intention doesn't include an elevated emotion, such as gratitude, savoring, joy (or something calming like "I feel peace and harmony" or "I feel relaxed"), then I encourage you to add these desired words into the mix here now, too. Write down yummy emotions that you *want* to feel, such as joy, peace, and gratitude.

....

....

....

....

....

....

If you can't access these emotions at all, thank you for being honest!

If this is the case for you, I invite you to make your New Moon intention as simple as this: *"The corners of my lips turn up as I start to feel joy."* This simple intention alone will change your life, if you follow all the Lunar Abundance steps at all the eight phases specified in this journal.

‹ Rewrite your New Moon intention here so it makes reference to elevated emotions:

....

....

....

....

....

....

....

....

....

....

....

....

....

....

....

....

....

....

Double-check your intention now.

- Is it all about you?

- Have you just set one intention, or have you tried to squish in an extra one?

- Is your intention framed in the positive (that is, what you are welcoming in, not what you are releasing at this time)?

- Does your intention contain elevated emotions that feel yummy and delicious? Can you feel your intention physically in your body?

❨ Make note now of any elements in your intention that you wish to remedy.

....

....

....

....

....

....

....

....

....

....

....

....

....

....

....

....

....

....

....

Your intention may have changed since your first draft above. That's perfect! That means that you are growing. Next up is your chance to draw it all together and declare your final New Moon intention.

MY FINAL NEW MOON INTENTION IS:

....

....

....

....

....

....

....

....

....

....

....

....

....

....

....

....

....

....

....

....

....

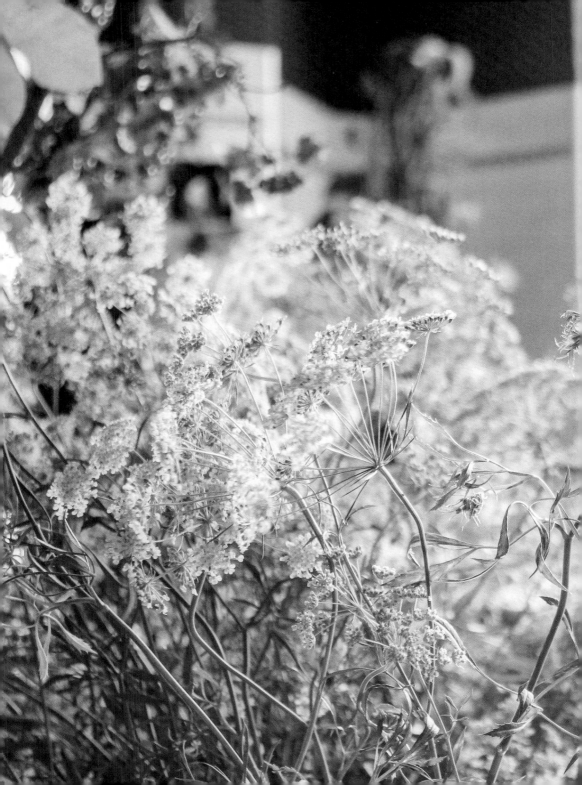

What in your *life* is *calling* for a new *perspective?*

WHAT HAPPENS NOW?

The next thing is to commit to using the exact wording of your intention, which you wrote above, as a trigger to return to the feeling of your intention, *every day*. But don't worry—it doesn't need to take up a ton of time every day! If you sit with your intention for just one minute a day throughout the entire Moon cycle, you will deeply nourish your intention.

The easiest way to cultivate a new habit like this is to simply add it to an existing one. For example, I meditate in the morning (in bed, because I'm lazy). So as soon as I wake up, I tune in to the feeling of my New Moon intention, before I even get out of bed. Rain, hail, or shine, I use my intention as a trigger and *feel it*. Just for a minute!

Because I encode my New Moon intention with juicy feelings and emotions, I *want* to feel it. Feeling good when I feel my intention is a powerful incentive for me to keep returning to this practice. The more I feel, the more my ability to feel increases. It's an upward spiral. It's natural and easy, it feels good, and repetition and consistency lead to excellent results.

If you don't meditate, then set up another trigger to return to your New Moon intention each day. For example, will you feel your intention when you brush your teeth, take a shower, start to cook dinner, or right before you go to sleep? Whatever it is for you, commit now to returning to your New Moon intention each day throughout the Moon cycle for one minute.

‹   When will you do this? Write that down here.

....

....

....

....

....

....

....

....

....

....

....

Now this is the final step, and it is a very important one. Take a moment to breathe, and rest your hand on your heart. Feel *grateful* that your New Moon intention is *already coming true*. Make sure you are feeling this gratitude—not just thinking about it. You will know you are feeling gratitude when the corners of your mouth turn up. If you are having trouble feeling grateful, return to what you wrote above about what is already working beautifully in your life. Anchor into this feeling, then return to your intention.

Don't worry about "how" it's going to happen yet. That comes later in the Moon cycle. For now, you are giving yourself the luxury of bathing in the *feeling*.

☾ Take a moment to record what that gratitude feels like in your body here. Get specific and name physical sensations and body parts (for example, warmth and tingling in your chest):

....

....

....

....

....

....

....

....

....

....

The reason we wrote down these words is they are very useful triggers for you to come back into your feeling each day through the Moon cycle ahead. You will return to this anchor of feeling grateful as your New Moon intention becomes a reality.

Now an important note: If you just read through the above prompts and thought about them, rather than writing down your responses, please go back through each of the steps and write down your answers. You won't "get it" until you unlock your Lunar Abundance journey with your writing.

Are you ready to carry on?

EXAMPLES OF NEW MOON INTENTIONS

Over time, I have come across many common mistakes in Lunar Abundance intention-setting. Below are some examples of New Moon intentions that may not work out very well because they don't align with the principles that I laid out for you above. If you see some variation of your intention among these, don't worry about it! I also offer suggestions on how to rework your intention so you get the best results.

Always revise with kindness. Remember, the cure, as ever, is always in the "problem." Your first draft is likely giving you valuable clues about how to proceed.

Also, remember that you can frame your lunar intention in whatever way you like. It's your intention! However, if you find that you are not getting results, then the invitation here is to review and consider if you could tweak your intention for a better outcome.

HEALTH AND DISCIPLINE

RATHER THAN: "I give up alcohol this Moon cycle."

RECOGNIZE: Your alcohol use may be affecting your health and relationships. You drink because your work is extremely stressful and wine at night calms you.

HOW ABOUT A NEW MOON INTENTION LIKE THIS: "I stand up strong at work, feeling calm and confident as I steer my team to resounding success with our current project." Or, "I feel healthy, vibrant, and well from head to toe as I nourish my temple with only that which serves me."

TRUE LOVE

RATHER THAN: "I want my husband to quit being so self-absorbed and show up for me again."

RECOGNIZE: You may be feeling rejected and out of control. You have a deep desire to feel safe, nurtured, and cared for.

HOW ABOUT A NEW MOON INTENTION LIKE THIS: "I feel joy in my heart as I co-create a mutually loving and supportive marriage."

YOUR FEELING SUPERPOWERS

RATHER THAN: "I literally cannot feel anything. I want to understand what I'm supposed to feel."

RECOGNIZE: You may have chosen to live from the neck up as a survival tactic. That was the best choice for you to make at a certain time to cope in your life, but it no longer serves you.

HOW ABOUT A NEW MOON INTENTION LIKE THIS: "I feel tingly in my hands as I gently open to feeling sensations of pleasure in my body."

PURPOSE AND PROSPERITY

RATHER THAN: "I want to make thousands with my essential oils business this month."

RECOGNIZE: You may hate your corporate job because you never wanted to do it, but you had to pay off your student loans. It stresses you out and you desperately want to escape the corporate grind and be like those goddesses online (seemingly) all having fun in Bali making six figures.

HOW ABOUT A NEW MOON INTENTION LIKE THIS: "I feel my whole body relax as I gratefully receive insight into my *true* soul purpose."

EMOTIONAL EXPLORATION

RATHER THAN: "I see golden light moving through me."

RECOGNIZE: You may still be captured by your thoughts, so dig a little deeper. Your thoughts are great, but emotions are self-revelatory. If you can't access your emotions at all, why not see what happens when you start to feel?

HOW ABOUT A NEW MOON INTENTION LIKE THIS: "I welcome warm feelings of peace and joy in my heart."

SIMPLICITY AS THE KEY TO ABUNDANCE

RATHER THAN: "I feel joy and excitement as I effortlessly create the life of my dreams this month, through finding the partner of my dreams, starting my own business (I plan to make a million dollars this year!), finding my dream home, and publishing my first children's book!"

RECOGNIZE: The top priority that feels most resonant for you this month may be just one of these. You might be rushing through your life, driven by beliefs about scarcity that you inherited, such as that you are not worthy of the markers of success you crave, or perhaps fear that if you don't do it all, *right now*, you might end up with nothing.

HOW ABOUT A NEW MOON INTENTION LIKE THIS: "I laugh with joy and I feel abundant throughout my body as I fulfill my dream of publishing, landing an agent to shop my manuscript to publishers this month."

—— SPIRAL UP! ——

RATHER THAN: "I mean, I still have no idea what my New Moon intention actually is. Figures. I've always been crap at stuff like this."

RECOGNIZE: The cure is in the problem! Make it really simple. You don't have access to your New Moon intention, even after journaling above? Then get out of your head now. This is the perfect time to practice being kind and loving to yourself.

HOW ABOUT A NEW MOON INTENTION LIKE THIS: "The corners of my mouth turn up as I joyfully welcome my New Moon intention."

—— CALM COHERENCE ——

RATHER THAN: My New Moon intention is *this*! Five minutes later— no, it's *this*! Next hour . . . in the morning . . . actually, wow, it's *this*! Day three . . . OMG now it's revealed itself to be *this*!

RECOGNIZE: While fine-tuning your intention may be part of the practice, being a cat-on-a-hot-tin-roof may be indicative of high anxiety and emotional reactivity. Think about what is going on under the surface of your life. Is it often tough for you to focus? What effect does this have on your life? How often do you allow yourself to pause, to rest, to practice being with the discomfort of what you are truly feeling?

HOW ABOUT A NEW MOON INTENTION LIKE THIS: "I breathe deeply and feel softness in my heart as I anchor into my soul medicine."

PEACE AND SOUL CONNECTION

RATHER THAN: "I feel happy as I use Instagram less this Moon cycle."

RECOGNIZE: You may be exhausted because you are not sleeping, because you can't stop scrolling until way past the time you meant to go to bed, and you have no time to think about how to cultivate genuine connection because the first thing you do in the morning is pick up your phone to turn off the alarm and react to what notifications came in overnight. Realize that you may be scrolling because you are addicted to technology that was designed to be addictive and keep you scrolling. The more you scroll, the more your life feels out of control, and it keeps snowballing until you are totally overwhelmed. So you keep scrolling.

HOW ABOUT A NEW MOON INTENTION LIKE THIS: "I feel enlivened throughout my whole body as I start welcoming in new friends in real life." Or, "I feel peace and joy in my heart as I bounce out of bed each morning, focused and well-rested."

REFLECTIONS

You will notice that all these examples speak to deeper motivations and desires. Lunar Abundance intentions all feel juicy, embodied, and delicious—and all open up the space for magic! It is not like goal-setting, and it's not about simple "Moon manifestations." This process of intention-setting is unique and powerful.

Lunar Abundance is a profound self-knowledge practice with the added benefit of helping you to create the life that you truly want to lead, here in the real world. If you show up for it, it will bring you home to yourself, and then start to unlock surprises for you.

The first step in this journey is simply to be open, honest, and real with yourself. The easiest way to start being real is to tune in to your top-level desires, senses, and feelings. This is how you access your subconscious, which encompasses most of your mind. We can't know ourselves, or our blind spots, until we delicately access our subconscious, and start to replace any old blocking beliefs hidden within, with new and creative beliefs.

The second element is treating whatever you find with love and kindness. You can see that there is no need to berate yourself about anything that you uncover in this practice. It is about being honest and *always* being kind and compassionate with yourself. And remember: Whatever you find is perfect for you right here, right now. There will always be a cure in the "problem" itself. Also, this early stage in the Moon cycle is not about the how you are going to make it happen.

The only decision that you need to make at this point? Simply decide to start the Lunar Abundance practice. Commit to it, for just one Moon cycle, and then honestly assess the results for yourself and see what is working.

Are you ready to commit to just one Moon cycle with Lunar Abundance?

Simple New Moon Ceremony

You may wish to create a beautiful New Moon ceremony—think candles, incense, and anything that stimulates your senses. The senses are the pathway out of the conscious mind, and into the subconscious. This is the purpose of a ceremony. But simple is good. You don't need to make it fancy. It's not about the candles and crystals. If they make you feel good, if they make you happy—go for it! The idea is to have fun and relax. If not, no worries. This is about your connection to *yourself*.

Here's an example:

1. On the next New Moon, prepare your sacred space. Activate your senses by lighting a candle, brewing a cup of herbal tea, and sitting on a comfortable cushion or rug.

2. Lay out this journal and a pen, close the door, and turn off your phone.

3. Close your eyes, place one hand on your heart and one on your belly to connect with your physical body, and breathe deeply. If you do this, there is no need to mentally work out what your intention is. Just see what feeling emerges in your body as you sit and breathe.

4. Now, ask yourself what you most desire, and wait to hear the answer. If there's something specific on your mind, ask for clarity on it.

5. Notice how the answer feels in your body. Do you feel tingles of excitement? Do you feel peace and expansion?

6. Tap into the power of elevated emotions by allowing yourself to feel grateful that you have already achieved your goal. Feel this in your body.

7. Open your eyes, and write down your intention to declare what you are creating.

(Refer back to the journaling prompts above for more suggestions on how to set an effective New Moon intention.)

Remember:

It can take some practice to get "into" your body, so don't worry if it doesn't happen right away. This takes practice! As you follow the Moon's cycles over time, your feelings will come more and more easily, until the process becomes effortless. It is like a muscle that keeps growing in strength.

As you will discover, so much more will become effortless, too . . .

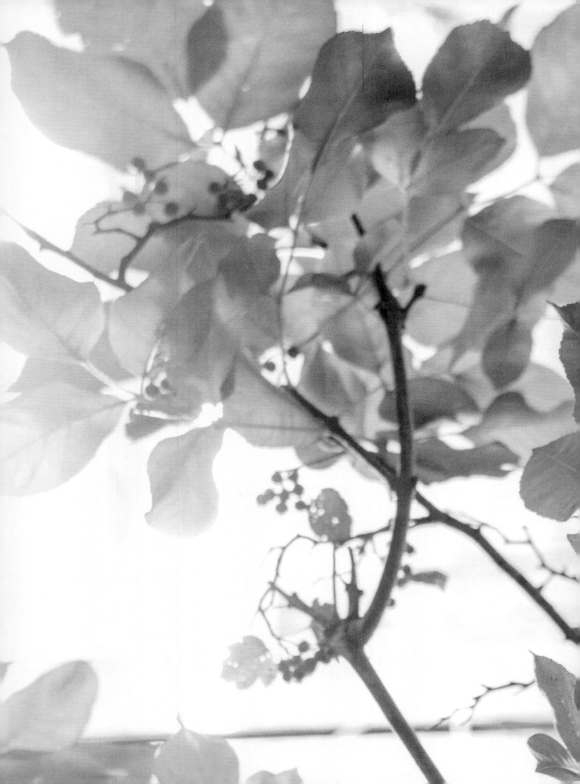

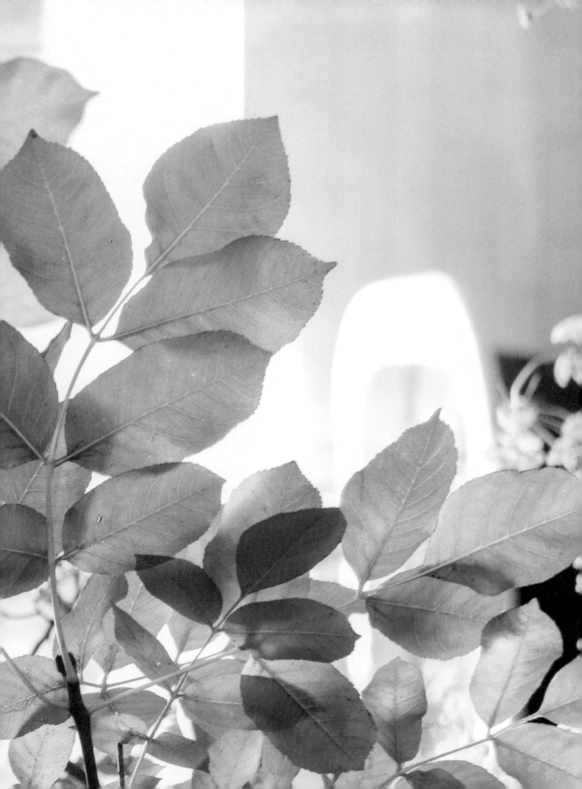

"Smile, breathe and
go slowly."

—*Thich Nhat Hanh*

Crescent Moon

☾

*"I relax into my intention.
I breathe."*

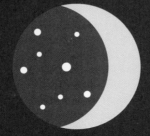

Lunar Abundance intention-setting encourages us to take personal responsibility for our lives and clarify what we really want. In the next phase, the Crescent Moon, we are introduced to a new element of the practice: the sacred marriage of *Doing* and *Being*.

By following the *Doing* and *Being* phases in this practice, you will become more healthy, calm, and relaxed, with more space for the priorities that you have identified as truly important for you, such as relating and connecting, health and well-being. A deep dive into *Doing* and *Being* is contained in my original *Lunar Abundance* book. This journal offers you a hint about these elements, to enable you to tap into their magic. In brief: The eight lunar phases are paired up. We will have a Doing phase, followed by a Being phase. The first, the New Moon, is a Doing phase (we actively set an intention together). Next is the Crescent Moon, and it is a Being phase. The pairs follow each other, so a Being phase will follow a Doing phase. After the Crescent Moon phase, we will have the First Quarter Moon phase, which is a Doing phase. Then the Gibbous Moon phase, another Being phase, and so on.

When it's a *Being* Moon phase, you have permission to take it a little easier.

When it's a *Doing* Moon phase, it's your nudge to get moving and make things happen.

Lunar Abundance offers a way to practice the dance between *Doing* and *Being*, an important skill for sustainable and fulfilling success. For me, the real magic is contained in the *Being* phases, because this is when we *feel*. To be clear, this is not about the Moon making us do anything, or making us feel a certain way. It's simply a guide for living in a sustainable way.

Here, we are working with the Moon as a natural timekeeper. What is helpful about linking *Doing* and *Being* to the Moon phases is that this linkage offers repetitive and predictable guidance for scheduling your life and work.

Rather than overscheduling yourself and getting exhausted, flaky, and burned out (over and over again), this practice offers a healthier, more realistic way to live.

The result? Over time, you build up a sustainable rhythm in life and work.

Before we go any further, I invite you to consider whether you are more *Doing*-oriented or more *Being*-oriented, in general.

If you are more *Doing*-oriented (like me!), you will likely find that, at first, introducing the *Being* phases will be more challenging, and then more rewarding (stop hustling your way to burnout, and then collapsing in a heap, time and time again).

If you are more *Being*-oriented, you will find that the *Doing* phases may help you to stop dreaming about the future—and actually make some things happen for yourself!

At the Crescent Moon phase, rather than diving right into further action and "making our intention happen," we get to practice Being.

Obviously, life does not stop in the Being phases. It all carries on, especially if you have people depending on you. But the energy shifts a little, and your process with your intention can shift, too. At a Being phase, the invitation is to be a little more reflective, introspective, and decide to "be" and feel more, rather than to "do" more. The journal prompts below will help you start to uncover what this might mean for you.

What does the Crescent Moon phase mean for your intention?

With the sliver of light that comes when the Crescent Moon is in the sky, we can start to see some greater clarity emerging around our intention in the external world. If so, this can be heartening, especially when our New Moon intention seemed a bit vague and unclear to us a few days ago. But it also can seem frustrating when just a little bit of clarity emerges, and we are ready to rock and roll with our intention.

When we have identified desires or preferences, the temptation for us is to launch into more of the "How can I make this happen?" energy right away—the scripting, the organizing, the mental categorizing. Believe me, I know! But, instead, the invitation for the next few days is just to relax.

To do this, sit with your intention in meditation every single day for at least one minute. Even in this Being phase, your intention is still cooking. Still *feel* the feeling of your intention each day, but don't strive to bring your intention to fruition right now. Just let it be.

This is practice for another way of being: learning how to create sustainable success in accordance with natural rhythms (and to cultivate greater abundance at the same time). I can't tell you what magic will unfold for you in these phases. I don't even know what magic will be revealed to *me*. This is part of the mystery (which, you'll recall, is part of the practice!).

You may be wondering how to "do" less and "be" more. Here are some quick tips on how to do just that (check out my *Lunar Abundance* book if you wish for more):

Over these next few days, indulge your senses: Take a luxurious soak in the bath, perhaps with flower petals. Give your legs a massage with some scented oil. Take a moment to notice and smell the roses—just because!

Enjoy a more passive breathing meditation, or yin yoga, rather than a more fiery practice.

Go for a walk, rather than a run or circuit training.

Don't push yourself to sprint, if you're not feeling the urge.

Be gentle. Be kind—to yourself.

Try receiving more. You may be presented with opportunities to practice receiving and, as you pay attention, this can play out in unexpected ways with your intention—ways that you would not even have been able to script if you had tried!

This may sound abstract, but when you follow the prompts below and notice what is happening in your world in this phase, you will start to find reference points in your own experience.

JOURNAL PROMPTS FOR THE CRESCENT MOON

For many who work with Lunar Abundance, the Being phases are a challenge. Why? Because we are so used to being applauded and awarded for doing things to achieve a particular goal. Yet, creating a natural shift in energy between Doing and Being will help you align with the natural flow of creative energy you are working with here.

❨ Consider what feelings and thoughts you associate with simply Being. (Lazy? Impatient? Natural?)

....

....

....

....

....

....

....

....

‹   What judgments do you make about simply Being? Are these really true? How might you awaken your curiosity about these judgments instead?

....
....
....
....
....
....
....
....
....
....
....

‹   How can you be gentle with yourself during this phase?

....
....
....
....
....
....
....
....
....
....
....
....

‹ As longtime Lunar Abundance practitioner Dr. Jennifer Mullan has suggested, do you have a "resistance to ease"? What might be some of the deeper reasons for this? Consider your family history, and other socio-cultural factors that may have influenced you in this regard.

....

....

....

....

....

....

....

....

....

....

‹ What might it feel like to allow greater ease in your life? What might you need to do differently?

....

....

....

....

....

....

....

....

❮ What could help your body (and expectations) to soften and relax now?

....
....
....
....
....
....
....
....
....
....
....

❮ How might you approach your life over the next few days from a Being perspective?

....
....
....
....
....
....
....
....
....
....
....

❨ How are you experiencing your intention in this first Being phase, the Crescent Moon?

....

....

....

....

....

....

....

....

....

....

....

❨ As you sit with your intention daily, what, if any, questions or realizations arise?

....

....

....

....

....

....

....

....

....

....

....

What will be revealed as you sink deeper into the Being of this practice is quite . . . magical.

Again, you can't just read the prompts above without actually doing the practice.

If you do that, the prompts will seem abstract and meaningless. Lunar Abundance is an experience, and you don't experience through reading. You read with your conscious mind. You experience through feeling. This journal is simply providing a portal for you to access raw experience.

For the best results with Lunar Abundance, show up like this:

1. Return to the *feeling* of your New Moon intention each day through-out the cycle.
2. Write out your answers to the prompts above and try the "activities."
3. Reflect on what starts to unfold with your intention as a result.

To anchor into this present moment, simply notice your breath. If life feels overwhelming right now, use your breath to soften into life.

You have permission to relax. How will you chill out (just a little) today?

....
....
....
....
....
....
....
....

....

....

....

....

....

....

....

....

....

....

We can choose abundance in this moment. We can choose presence in the next breath. This is your invitation to breathe deeply and gently relax into your day.

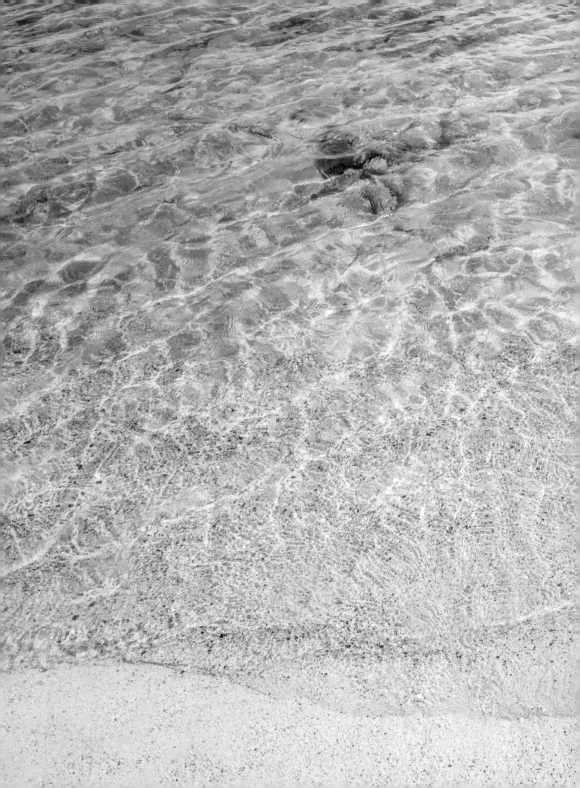

"Essentialism is not about how to get more things done, it's about how to get the right things done. It doesn't mean just doing less for the sake of doing less either. It is about making the wisest possible investment of your time and energy in order to operate at your highest point of contribution by doing only what is essential."

—Greg McKeown

First Quarter Moon

☽

"I take discerning action to
support my intention."

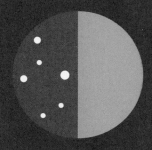

Welcome to another Doing phase. As the Moon waxes to full, you may find that some more "Doing" energy starts to flow through your life and work over the next few days. And if you've been doing the inner work over the past week, you will likely notice that things start to move with your intention. You may notice changes in your external world—and these will more than likely follow shifts in your inner landscape.

You may start to be presented with opportunities to take *action*. It is important to manage your expectations with this, though. It is not that your intention will suddenly become real at this stage (although, if it does—fabulous!). The Lunar Abundance technique is a slow and gentle process. It is not a one-lunar-cycle practice. You will find that cultivating abundance is best practiced at a relaxed and graceful pace. The trick is to notice—and be grateful for—the opportunities for minor action over the next few days.

You may be presented with small opportunities to take action at first. But even these little steps will give you the opportunity to find out more about your intention, and what it will take to come to fruition.

Take *discerning* action.

Discernment is key in this practice. And the First Quarter Moon phase is the perfect time to practice taking discerning action.

Just because you are presented with a particular opportunity doesn't mean that it is a sign that you should go down a particular path. Yes, it might be. But it also might be a sign that it's time for you to be very clear about who you are, what you want, what it's going to take to bring it to fruition, and why you want it. You don't need to take every opportunity for action at this stage. The decision not to take action may can be just as important. There is an abundance of opportunity for you.

Caveat: If you are someone who finds it difficult to take any action at all, be mindful about using this advice as an excuse. Pay close attention to what is happening in your life over the next few days, and notice the minor actions in front of you that you could take.

But if you are someone who is prone to seizing every opportunity in front of you, ask yourself over the next few days whether you could, perhaps, be more conscious about which actions you take. Cultivate discernment at the First Quarter Moon phase.

JOURNAL PROMPTS FOR THE FIRST QUARTER MOON

Many who are new to the Lunar Abundance practice particularly relish the First Quarter Moon Phase. This is the time to take action to support your lunar intention. You will be presented with opportunities—or you'll make opportunities happen—where you can take discerning action to support your lunar intention, but always remember that discerning action is key.

‹   So what actions could you take at this stage?

....

....

....

....

....

....

....

....

....

....

....

....

....

....

....

....

❮ Which of these actions feel aligned with your intention for this Moon cycle?

....

....

....

....

....

....

....

....

....

....

....

....

....

....

....

....

....

....

❨ What *one* mindful, discerning action will you take in this phase?

....

....

....

....

....

....

....

....

....

....

....

....

....

....

❮ Return here afterward to reflect. How did you feel after taking this action?

....

....

....

....

....

....

....

....

....

....

....

....

....

....

❮ What were the results of taking this action?

....

....

....

....

....

....

....

....

....

....

....

....

....

....

....

....

....

....

....

....

....

....

....

....

❨ How would life feel if you cut your to-do list in half? Be discerning. What is most important? And what is just filler? You have the power to choose.

....

....

....

....

....

....

....

....

....

....

....

....

....

....

....

....

‹ Choose wisely. What do you stand for? Let your actions speak loudly today.

....

....

....

....

....

....

....

....

....

....

....

....

....

....

....

....

....

....

....

....

....

Sometimes you take the best action by choosing not to go through with it. Only you can make the call. Look within for the answer.

"If you trust in Nature, in the small things that hardly anyone sees and that can so suddenly become huge, immeasurable; if you have this love for what is humble and try very simply, as someone who serves, to win the confidence of what seems poor, then everything will become easier for you."

—Rainer Maria Rilke

Gibbous Moon

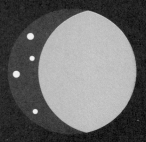

"*I trust that the perfect
intention is coming into form
at the perfect time.*"

The Gibbous Moon phase is another Being phase. It is now time to reflect on the actions that you took in the First Quarter Moon phase, and give yourself time to process the effects of these actions. It is now time to shift out of hunting energy and start to *trust* yourself—and the process.

You may find that some questions start to emerge at the Gibbous phase. For example, you might start to wonder:

What does it really mean to create a life of abundance?

What kind of changes will be required in your life to allow your intention to come into being? Are you actually ready to make these changes?

Listen to yourself and trust your own answers. You are the expert on you!

This can be challenging when we have been trained to be told what to do—by marketing and advertising, by social media, by politicians, by opinionated leaders and people in our life.

However, Lunar Abundance invites you to create more self-sovereignty.

This journal offers you the guidance to discover your sense of self. It's a way to start to wind yourself back to you, but the only person who can ultimately find you is you. The Gibbous Moon phase is the perfect time to start to understand which desires are emanating from a deep urge to evolve your soul—and not from the grasping of your ego. You can gently expand beyond your limitations. But you don't need to do it just in one lunar cycle.

There is no need to put your mind to work to ascertain your limitations. Instead, return to and focus on the feelings that you accessed in the New Moon phase. (You will see now that this is one of the reasons elevated emotions are so important.) Keep meditating each day with your intention—for at least one minute. Use the words from your New Moon intention as triggers to come back to the warm and yummy feeling that you created.

Keep sinking into the feeling—anchoring into the physical sensations in your body. When you are connected with this intention, it is easier to expand, slowly, beyond your limitations.

The invitation at this lunar phase is to *trust*:

To trust your own personal process.

To trust that you can move at whatever pace you choose.

To trust that it is safe to tiptoe into a life of greater abundance.

JOURNAL PROMPTS FOR THE GIBBOUS MOON

Reflecting on the actions you took during the First Quarter Moon phase can summon feelings of doubt, uncertainty, or impatience.

‹ What would it feel like to approach these emotions with curiosity at this time?

....

....

....
....
....
....
....
....
....
....
....
....
....
....

‹ Have you been invited to trust at this lunar phase? What did that look like?

....
....
....
....
....
....
....
....
....
....
....
....
....
....

....

....

....

....

....

....

....

❨ What does trust feel like in your body? What physical clues signal this state?

....

....

....

....

....

....

....

....

....

....

....

....

....

....

....

....

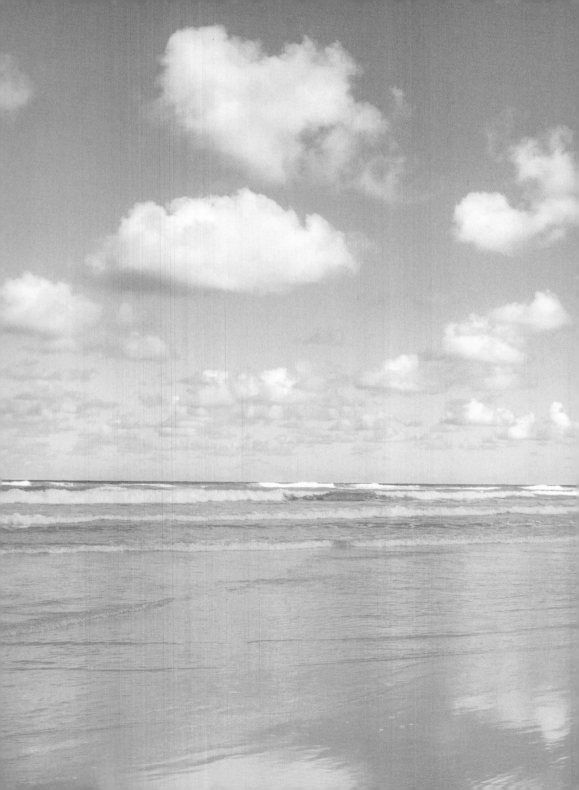

Will you *stretch*
beyond your doubts?
Can you *soften* into a
state of *Trust?*

❮ How do you feel now about the action you took at the First Quarter Moon phase?

....
....
....
....
....
....
....
....
....
....
....
....
....

❮ What questions have arisen about what it may take to bring your intention to fruition?

....
....
....
....
....
....
....
....

‹ What emotions are arising for you right now? Name these with specificity.

‹ If you are feeling uncomfortable with these emotions, do you notice yourself reaching for a distraction? What are you reaching for? Remember, the more you allow yourself to simply be with uncomfortable emotions, the more present and attuned to yourself you become.

‹ Can you turn around any emotions? (Return to the New Moon section above for more on this.) Remember, the cure is always in the "problem."

....
....
....
....
....
....
....
....
....
....
....
....
....
....
....
....
....
....
....
....
....
....

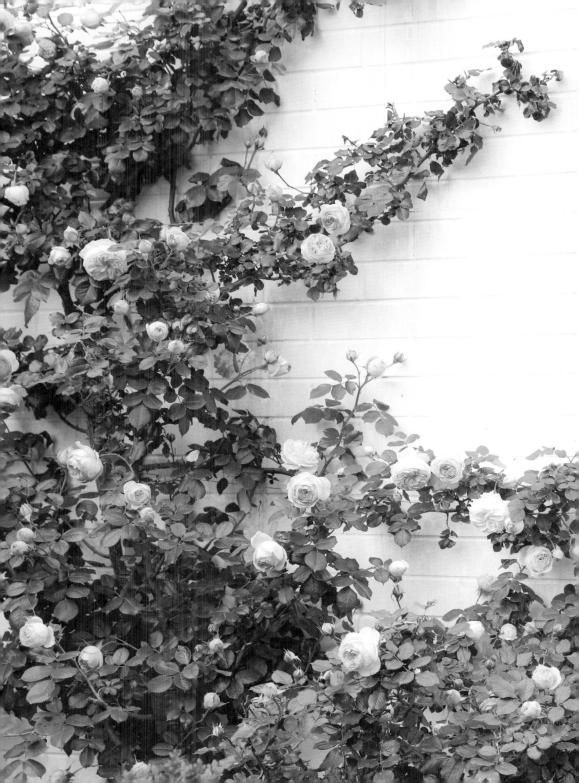

Trust. You are
transforming. Your *soul*
knows the *way.*

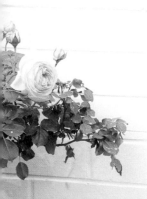

If you are struggling with this phase, take a moment to reflect: Where else in your life do you find it challenging to take your hands off the wheel of control and just let things . . . be?

‹ Imagine what could be different in your life if you could allow yourself to trust in the absence of immediate validation or instant gratification? What possibilities might open up?

....
....
....
....
....
....
....
....
....
....
....
....
....
....
....
....
....
....
....
....
....
....
....

‹ If you've sat in the "fire" of trust for a day or so (which can be hard!), what has happened inside you? Remember: There's rarely growth without discomfort, and the more we practice feeling and being okay with discomfort, the greater our potential for expansion into abundance.

....

....

....

....

....

....

....

....

....

....

....

....

....

....

....

....

....

....

....

....

....

❮ How do you feel you know yourself more now, after undertaking these reflections?

....
....
....
....
....
....
....
....
....
....
....
....
....
....
....
....
....
....
....
....
....
....
....
....

❰ You are not locked into a contract with the intention that you set at the New Moon. If you realize during this phase that your intention is too big, or the adjustments that it will require are too much for you right now, take some time to adjust your intention now. Does your intention still feel right for you or do you wish to tweak it?

....

....

....

....

....

....

....

....

....

....

....

....

....

....

....

....

....

....

....

....

....

....

◑ This is a Being phase, and it has been a very internal time. However, take a moment to reflect: What do you see happening with your intention in your external world? How do you feel about that?

....

....

....

....

....

....

....

....

....

....

....

....

....

....

....

....

....

....

....

....

....

....

"I'm learning to love the sound
of my feet walking away from
things not meant for me."

—*Author Unknown*

Full Moon

☽

"I move ahead with my intention now" Or, *"I accept that my intention was not for the best at this time. I release it, and course-correct."*

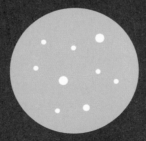

Go outside this evening. Look up. Are you seeing a gorgeous Full Moon? This is the lunar phase where the Moon is far-thest from the Sun, and the face of the Moon is reflecting the light of the Sun onto the Earth. There's a lot of light under the Full Moon (especially if you are outside in nature at this time!).

Much is visible for you in relation to your intention right now—if you look around. This is the point at which it will be abundantly clear whether you are on the right track. And, if it is not right, this is the perfect time to course-correct.

If you overstretched with your original intention, if you are finding that there is too much pressure on you, now is the time to notice this, and now is the time to detach from your intention. Let it go. Feel gratitude for what has already come to pass.

You can go deeper again in the next lunar cycle. It bears repeating: This is not a one-cycle process. The Moon is the essence of abundance. There's another lunar cycle starting again in a couple of weeks.

Releasing an intention is not a failure. Trial and error is how you build trust in the world and in yourself. This us how, ultimately, you will get to know yourself in a much more intimate and loving way. This is the way you start to more deeply understand the evolution of your soul, and not just the grasping wants of your mind or ego.

If you stopped working with your intention in this lunar cycle, be sure to come back to your intention now. Sit with it during a few minutes of meditation each day. If you *are* on the right track, you will start to see results from your intention now. That doesn't mean your intention will have been fully realized. That depends on how ambitious your intention was, and also whether you have done the necessary inner work. But if you have been doing the work, your next steps will be obvious now.

To open the space for abundance, you must be able to release, rather than hoard. It sounds simple, but requires practice. This may involve decluttering your desk or your closet. But even if you do not hoard physical things, you may be hoarding emotions and limiting beliefs about your worth, and fears about what may happen if you actually let go of those old beliefs that are keeping you small and "safe."

When you let go, you create space to welcome in so much more that is aligned with your true soul purpose, and with your continued growth and expansion.

Everything changes, all the time, and we must flow with this to attract abundance.

Note that this is a different concept than just spending all you have, or being flippant about what you receive. This is not what I mean by "letting go." When you truly have an abundant mind-set, you are not prone to excess; you live a simple life, and you cherish what you receive.

One way to practice this at the Full Moon phase is to allow the "light" of the Moon to illuminate what you are holding on to. Write down what you need to release on a piece of paper, and then burn that paper.

Also make a list of everything for which you forgive yourself—or that which you forgive others for. Then, burn the piece of paper and liberate yourself.

If you do these exercises by candlelight, it may feel like a lovely ritual. Or, allow yourself to think about what you want to release and then go running, dancing, swimming, take a shower. Shake it off—release it into the water!

JOURNAL PROMPTS FOR THE FULL MOON

The Full Moon is another Doing phase, which means it's a perfect time for action.

‹ In terms of the intention you set two weeks ago, what is clear to you at this phase?

....

....

....

....

....

....

....

....

....

....

....

....

....

....

....

....

....

At the light of the Full Moon, everything is illuminated—including your intention. It's also a time to release any unreasonable expectations you have about your intention. This is crucial. To allow our deepest desires to come into form, we have to learn to let go of whatever isn't in our best interest at this time, or to the attachments we carry about *how* our intentions come to fruition. What do you need to release? What will you let go of?

....

....

....

....

....

....

....

....

....

....

....

....

....

....

....

....

....

....

....

Let the *light* of the *Full Moon*
be your potent reminder to
let go of that which *no longer*
serves you.

....

....

....

....

....

....

....

....

....

....

....

....

‹ What did you learn in this Full Moon phase?

....

....

....

....

....

....

....

....

....

....

....

....

....

....

....

....

....

....

....

....

....

....

....

❮   What surprised you in this phase? What delighted you?

....

....

....

....

....

....

....

....

....

....

....

....

....

....

....

....

....

....

....

....

‹ After you do the Full Moon ceremony below, consider this: How are you feeling now?

....

....

....

....

....

....

....

....

....

....

....

....

....

....

....

....

....

....

....

❮ What is the one next step that you will take to make your intention come true?

....
....
....
....
....
....
....
....
....
....
....
....
....
....
....
....
....
....
....
....
....
....
....

Simple Full Moon Ceremony

Remember that a core principle of Lunar Abundance is connection. The Full Moon is the perfect time to tap into the principles of abundance and connection with others by celebrating our strengths. Here is a simple Full Moon ceremony that you may wish to try:

1. Bring two or three friends together on the day of the Full Moon. (It does not need to be at the exact time because Lunar Abundance is a guidance system; I do not suggest that the Moon "makes us" do anything.) You may wish to invite your friends to an afternoon in the park or to your house for a meal.

2. Prepare two pieces of paper and a pen for each person, a large bowl, and a lighter.

3. When you are together, ask each of them to write down the intention they are working to bring to life on the first piece of paper.

4. On the second piece of paper, ask them to write down whatever is holding them back from realizing this intention. What is keeping you languishing, rather than flourishing? For example, if you are afraid of being judged if you step out and become more visible by writing a book, write that down.

5. One at a time, ask each person to read their intention aloud, and share what is keeping them from moving forward. Then, have each of them burn the second piece of paper in the bowl, while identifying a specific action that they will take to move toward their intention.

6. As each person burns their list, ask the other group members to identify and affirm a strength of the person who is burning the paper. Each group member could state this in turn. For example, one group member may look toward the person burning the paper, and state, "I see your courage to be seen as who you really are."

7. Repeat the ceremony so that each person has publicly declared their intentions, burned their fears, identified a specific action they will take to move forward and flourish, and felt their strength affirmed.

8. Consider checking in with each of the participants at the end of the ceremony to ensure that they are all feeling complete and fulfilled. If one of them is not, you may wish to ask that person what support they need, and provide that support. Remember that support may not be in you giving them your analysis and advice. Let the person in question identify the specific support that they need in that moment, listen, and respond accordingly (checking in again at the end to ensure that they feel complete).

Remember:

Abundance is not about accumulating more "stuff." It's the courage to dream bigger, to trust that you are worthy of creating a better life, and to believe that you will be supported to flourish if you set the right goals, show up to support others, and do the work.

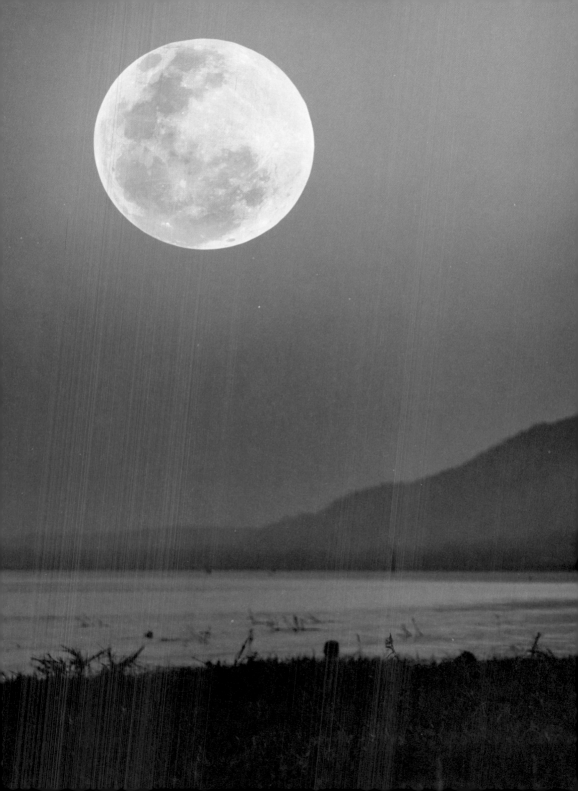

You can *release* your *fears* in order to gracefully *expand* and *awaken*.

"Let gratitude be the pillow upon which you kneel to say your nightly prayer. And let faith be the bridge you build to overcome evil and welcome good."

—*Maya Angelou*

Disseminating Moon

"I feel grateful that my
intention is coming into form
in the perfect way. I receive
with gratitude."

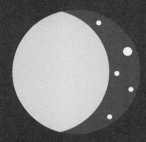

Another Being phase is upon us. It is time to joyfully receive what has come into your life, and any transformation in your inner world that has occurred since you set a New Moon intention a couple of weeks ago. The key to receiving is the practice of *gratitude*. Pay particular attention to your gratitude practice over the next few days.

It may be that what has come into your life since the New Moon, and the shifts you have made, became abundantly clear under the light of the Full Moon. Or you may be wondering why your intention hasn't come to pass, and why others seem to be more committed to theirs or having more success than you. If you are feeling frustrated, this is the ideal moment for you to pause, journey within, and notice any changes—however small—that have occurred in your life since the New Moon.

It may not all be fireworks and roses when you first start out working with this practice. That's okay. This will help you to cultivate patience and awareness. The trick is to start to notice the subtle shifts in this lunar cycle. The paradox is that the more that you feel grateful for tiny, almost imperceptible shifts, and the more you start to receive the small gifts, the bigger and faster changes come into your life.

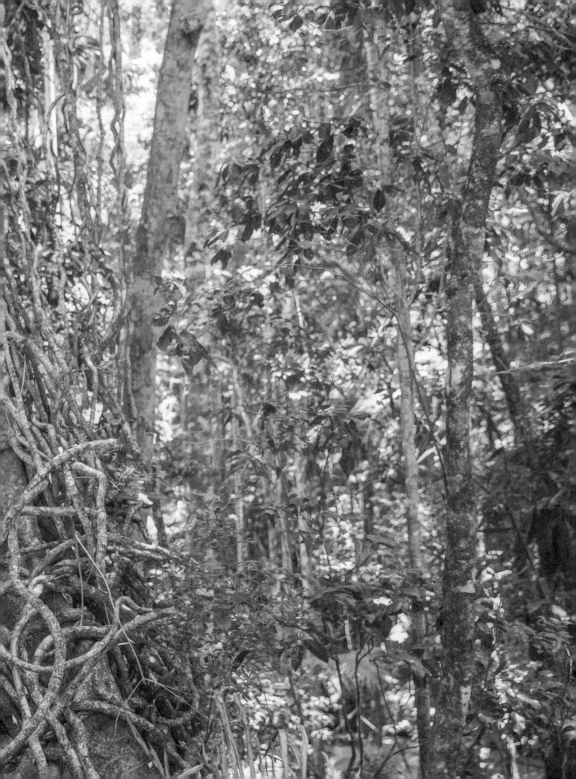

❮ What is coming into your life with your intention now?

....
....
....
....
....
....
....
....
....
....
....
....
....
....
....
....
....
....
....
....
....
....
....
....
....

᚜ How might you savor or celebrate what you are receiving now?

....
....
....
....
....
....
....
....
....
....
....
....
....
....
....

᚜ This is another Being phase. How does this feel for you, at this time, compared to how you felt in the Gibbous Moon phase?

....
....
....
....
....
....

....

....

....

....

....

....

❨ What do you notice about how you are relating to the concept of Being
and Doing since you started this Lunar Abundance practice?

....

....

....

....

....

....

....

....

....

....

....

....

....

....

....

....

....

....

❨ There is great power in gratitude. If you're in a difficult situation, changing your mindset alone won't make your troubles vanish, but gratitude *will* help you see the next step that you can take, and it will infuse you with optimism and confidence. So, what are you grateful for? What will you receive with genuine gratitude today?

....

....

....

....

....

....

....

....

....

....

....

....

....

....

....

....

....

....

....

Lunar Loves, it is safe to receive! A grateful life is a full life. Share your gratitude and allow it to expand.

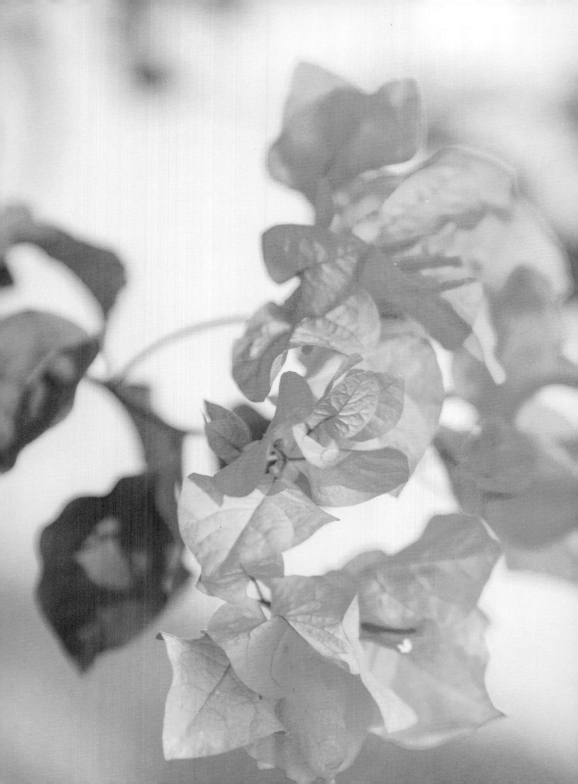

"If we are stretching to live wiser and not just smarter, we will aspire to learn what love means, how it arises and deepens, how it withers and revives, what it looks like as a private good but also as a common good."

—*Krista Tippett*

Third Quarter Moon

☾

*"Now that I am receiving my
intention, I give back from a
place of abundance."*

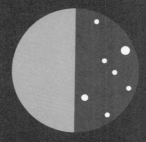

So far our focus has been on what you want to bring into your life, and the adjustments that you are making to your own mind-set to attract them. This is the necessary precursor to abundance—filling up your own tank, so to speak, so you are able to then help others. At this lunar phase, we shift the emphasis to consider how to *give*.

The more you have, the more you can give.

In this, the final Doing stage of the lunar cycle, consider how you can give value to others from a place of abundance, inspiration, and high energy. Abundant giving may sound simple, but it can take practice. The important principles for this phase are:

1. Give genuinely, without expecting to receive.

2. Give generously.

But:

3. Consider not giving because you feel obliged to. Or, consider whether it is just your habitual pattern to give and give.

For instance, you might give because you feel this is the only way that you will be liked or respected, or because you find it too difficult to receive.

4.   If your tank is empty, consider giving to yourself first.

Over time you will start to identify your own giving patterns. Make note of this. Be a detective, investigating yourself. Remember that you have more lunar cycles ahead to help you shift this, if you determine that you need to. Old patterns may shift slowly. The trick is not to stress out, and not to try to "fix" yourself.

Just notice what is going on for you, and allow yourself to accept and love what you find. And, over the next few days, identify an opportunity where you are able to give generously—from a place of abundance.

How can you tell when you are giving from a place of abundance? Because of how it *feels*. If you feel energized when you think about giving, and if you feel fantastic afterward, then you are giving from a place of abundance.

If you feel exhausted and drained, that's okay. Ask yourself whether you had a choice *not* to give in that particular situation. Remember: It's *okay* not to give sometimes. You do not need to feel guilty. You definitely do not need to push yourself to give if you are too exhausted and depleted to do so. This is how you develop boundaries. And it is how you can cultivate the practice of abundant giving.

Of course, sometimes you just *do* need to give, no matter what. If you have people in your life who depend on you for essentials, such as food and personal care, then adjust this lunar phase practice for your situation. In this case, think about how you could make minor adjustments to your giving. Could you pace yourself a little more? Are you giving a little more than necessary? Could you speak to a family member to bring in a little extra support? Could you start to consider a more long-term arrangement that will support your staying healthy and happy moving forward?

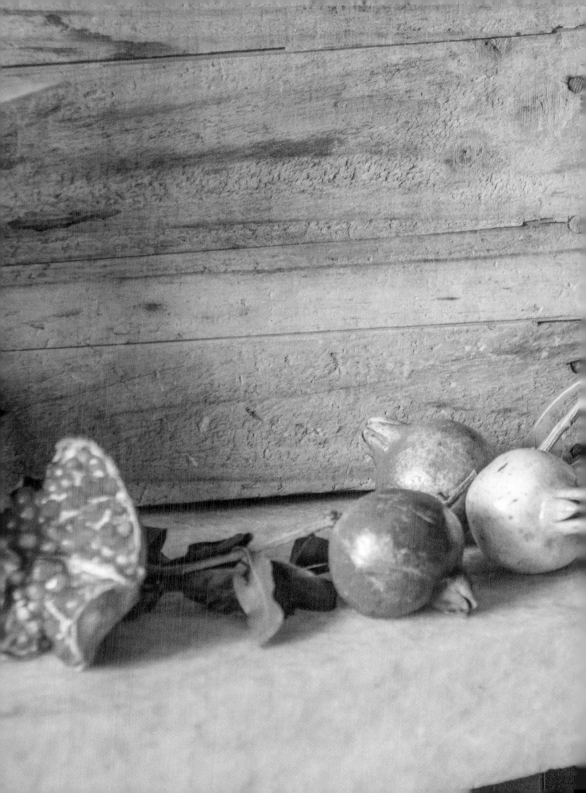

How can you be *generous*? With your *time*? With your *energy*? With your *love*? *Giving* doesn't always have to be *material*.

Even minor adjustments at this lunar phase can result in profound changes in your life.

JOURNAL PROMPTS FOR THE THIRD QUARTER MOON

At this Third Quarter Moon phase, we are invited to give from a full cup. When we give from a place of abundance we don't feel drained—giving feels joyous and delicious. So, if you feel that you need to, you can choose to give to yourself during this cycle. This phase may highlight features of your giving pattern. Observe closely.

   ‹   When you think about giving at this phase, what comes up for you?

....
....
....
....
....
....
....
....
....
....
....
....
....
....
....

‹ Will you choose to give to yourself at this phase? Or give to others?

....
....
....
....
....
....
....
....
....
....
....
....
....
....
....
....
....
....
....
....
....
....
....
....
....

❮ What have you noticed about your giving patterns? Are you giving because you feel you should? Or does it feel natural to give to others?

....

....

....

....

....

....

....

....

....

....

....

....

....

....

....

....

....

....

....

....

....

....

....

How does it feel in your body when you give from a full cup?

....

....

....

....

....

....

....

....

....

....

....

....

....

....

....

....

....

....

....

....

....

....

‹ If you don't feel as if you are giving from a full cup, but you feel compelled to give anyway, why might you be doing this?

....

....

....

....

....

....

....

....

....

....

....

‹ What might you change in future?

....

....

....

....

....

....

....

....

....

....

◖ What is happening with your intention now? Do you need to take further action to make it a reality?

....
....
....
....
....
....
....
....
....
....
....
....
....
....
....
....
....
....
....
....
....
....
....

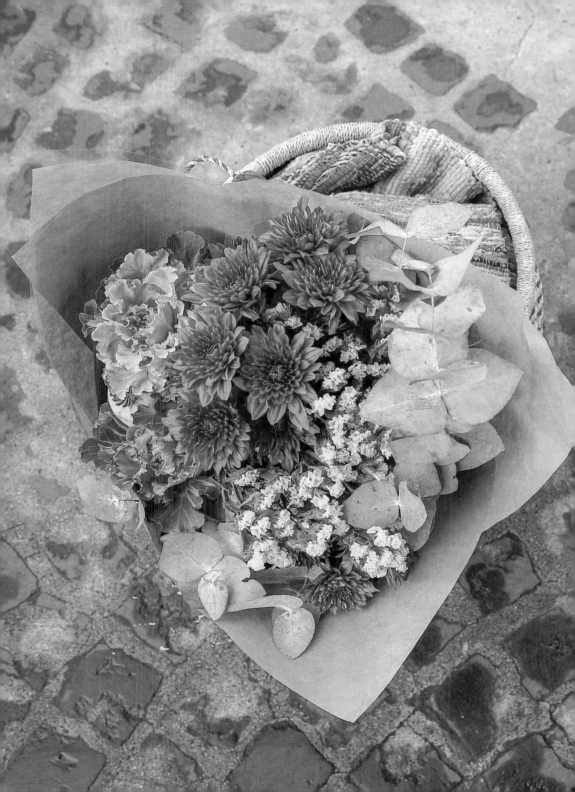

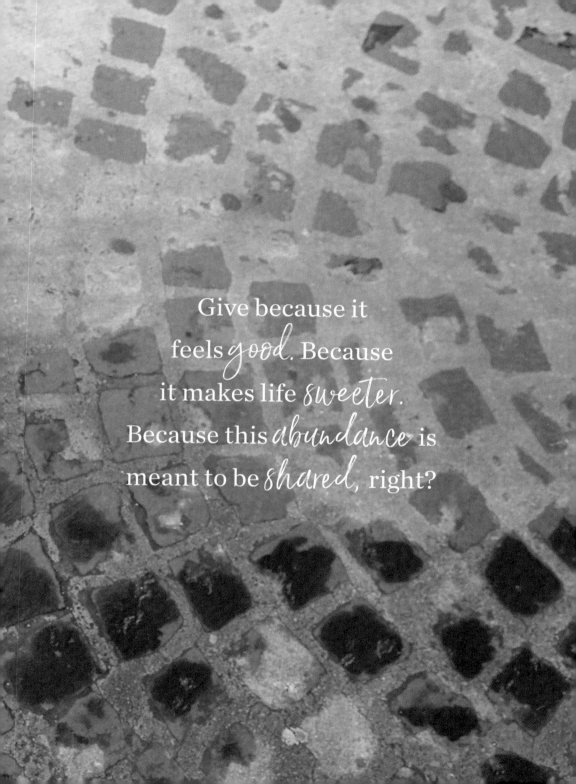

Give because it
feels *good*. Because
it makes life *sweeter*.
Because this *abundance* is
meant to be *shared*, right?

"Not what we have, but
what we enjoy, constitutes
our abundance."

—*Epicurus*

Balsamic Moon

☾

"I reflect with thanks. I rest.
I restore."

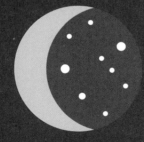

This is the final phase of the lunar cycle. If you lost track this month, please do not worry! The lunar phases repeat with each lunar cycle, so you will be able to share, ask questions, and work through any unfinished business in the next lunation. If you have followed along on this lunar cycle, this is a time to really s-l-o-w down. The Balsamic Moon phase is the ultimate Being time.

This is a time for reflection on what has come to pass in your life over the past lunar month, to reflect back on your original New Moon intention, to reflect on each phase from this cycle, and to consider where you were at the start and where you are now.

Rather than leaping forward to the next shiny object or the new thing (or the next New Moon intention!), the invitation now is to be more mindful about what has *actually* happened in your life this past month, and allow this growing self-awareness to guide where you want to go next. This is how we start to strip back the layers of conditioning in our world and start to understand who we really are. This is how we come into closer relationship with our true soul purpose, and our real reason for being in the world.

The interesting thing is that our view of our progress at any given time is not always aligned with reality. It can feel as if we're going nowhere. But when we take a moment to pause and review our intention, and how it is unfolding, we can see that we've actually made huge progress in just a month.

Or, it can feel like things are happening like "magic," but that was simply the result of being very careful in creating your own map, course-correcting if more information came to light, and consistently showing up to your dreams each day by using your intention as a compass (and by returning to the feeling of it, just for a minute, each day).

A lovely practice now can be to return to your New Moon journal section to review what you wrote a month ago. Then, review your notes from the other phases now, too. What were your feelings? Your doubts? Your fears? Your worries? Your challenges? Your hopes and dreams? What were your small wins along the way? What did you learn? Rather than beat yourself up for doing something wrong, practice self-compassion. What might you do differently next time? How will you grow? As we know, the cure is always in the "problem."

Down the road, you may wish to return to your own Moon journals over time. How did you feel at the last Balsamic Moon phase? How about three Moons ago? How about last year?

The Moon cycle represents the essence of abundance. She never runs out! This is one of the reasons I still follow this practice after more than a decade. It just keeps going. It continues to bring so much richness and delight to my life, Moon cycle after Moon cycle, year after year. I still set my New Moon intentions, and I still sit with these intentions each day, because I have never found another personal growth practice that is so powerful and transformative, and yet feels so *good*.

Now, you'll recall that this practice is not about simply "improving." Lunar Abundance is about cultivating joy, peace, and purpose. So consider these questions at the Balsamic Moon phase: How might you cultivate joy? How might you celebrate?

Once you have reviewed your month during the Balsamic Moon phase, the hope is for you to experience gratitude for all that you have received, and all the ways you have grown this Moon cycle.

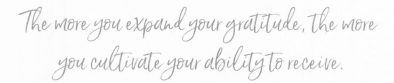

The more you expand your gratitude, the more you cultivate your ability to receive.

Also, the more you will be able to expand your ability to hold on to whatever you receive. Receiving abundance in your life is one thing. Being able to keep that abundance in your life is quite another. Through following this magical practice, we expand our receptivity in a sustainable way. We are doing this by carefully changing our belief systems so that we feel worthy and deserving of all that we need to live life in the most joyful and purposeful way. And this is what you will practice, over time, in upcoming lunar cycles.

For now, give yourself a pat on the back for following through on your first cycle! If you are reading this, it means that you have shown up for yourself, and for your dreams, in a way that most people never do. You have just set yourself apart from the rest—and I know that means you are well on your way to transforming your life, so you live with greater ease and flow by the Moon cycle.

Welcome to the Lunar Abundance family!

JOURNAL PROMPTS FOR THE BALSAMIC MOON

The Balsamic Moon phase is the most *Being* phase. It is a time to fully reflect on everything that has come into your life since you set your New Moon intention. On reflection, you may be surprised at the abundance that you have received.

‹ What has come into your life since the New Moon?

....

....

....

....

....

....

....

....

....

....

....

....

❮ What has happened in your life, and how can you link this back to your intention? Take the time to write this out—you may well be surprised!

....

....

....

....

....

....

....

....

....

....

....

....

....

....

....

....

....

....

❬ Did you sit with your intention each day for just one minute? If so, what happened? If you didn't, why did you stop? How might you do that differently in the next Moon cycle?

....

....

....

....

....

....

....

....

....

....

....

....

....

....

....

....

‹ If you haven't received everything that you desired yet, why do you think that might be? Are you celebrating what did come into your life, even if it was not necessarily what you expected?

....

....

....

....

....

....

....

....

....

....

....

‹ What did you learn through this process?

....

....

....

....

....

....

....

....

....

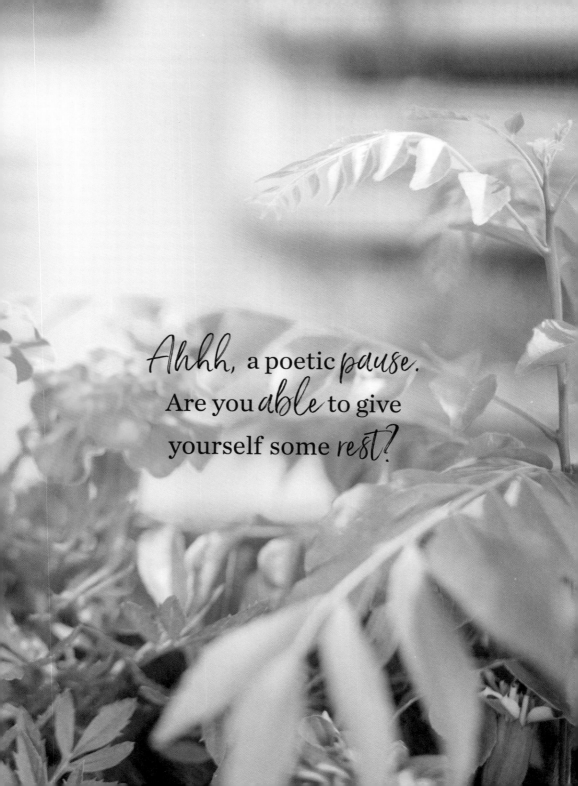

Ahhh, a poetic *pause.* Are you *able* to give yourself some *rest?*

....

....

....

....

....

....

....

‹ What might you do differently in the next Moon cycle?

....

....

....

....

....

....

....

....

....

....

....

....

....

....

....

◖ What has this brought to the surface for you? What would you like to deepen in future Moon cycles?

....

....

....

....

....

....

....

....

....

....

....

....

....

....

....

....

....

....

....

....

....

....

....

‹   What do you feel grateful for?

‹ Has the experience of gratitude shifted for you in this practice? Where do you *feel* it?

....
....
....
....
....
....
....
....
....
....
....
....
....
....
....
....
....
....
....
....
....
....
....

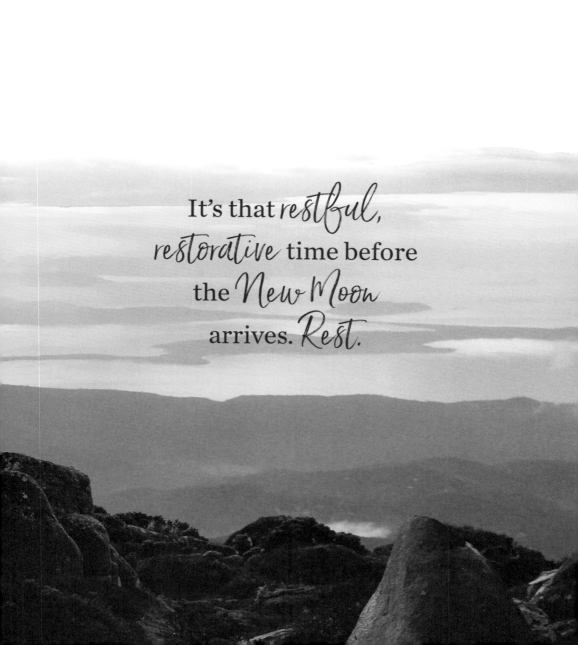

It's that *restful*, *restorative* time before the *New Moon* arrives. *Rest*.

CONCLUSION

This brings us to the end of the lunar cycle. This is not, however, the end of the Lunar Abundance practice. Again, the Moon cycle is the essence of abundance—it literally never runs out! The lunar cycle is very observable, trackable, and it repeats. We always have another chance in the next lunar cycle.

And if you really did the work? Well, it is time to layer your next New Moon intention onto what you have experienced in your life during this lunar cycle.

Once one lunar cycle concludes, this is not the "end" of that theme. We carry on, moving forward, continue to evolve, and *integrate* that theme in our lives, all the while.

If you would like to go deeper into this practice, please pick up a copy of my *Lunar Abundance* book, which is chock-full of more examples, case studies, resources, summaries, and journal prompts, to help you create your own dream life. It is available wherever books are sold.

Please also check out my website, LunarAbundance.com, which has plenty of free audio downloads, charts, and other resources to support you on your lunar journey.

The question now is . . .

What is your New Moon intention?

....
....
....
....
....
....
....
....
....
....
....
....
....
....
....
....
....
....
....
....
....
....

By the way, Lunar Loves, when you are on your second cycle (and beyond!), it is absolutely okay for you to repeat your intention from the last Moon cycle.

It's all about what feels most resonant for you at the time!

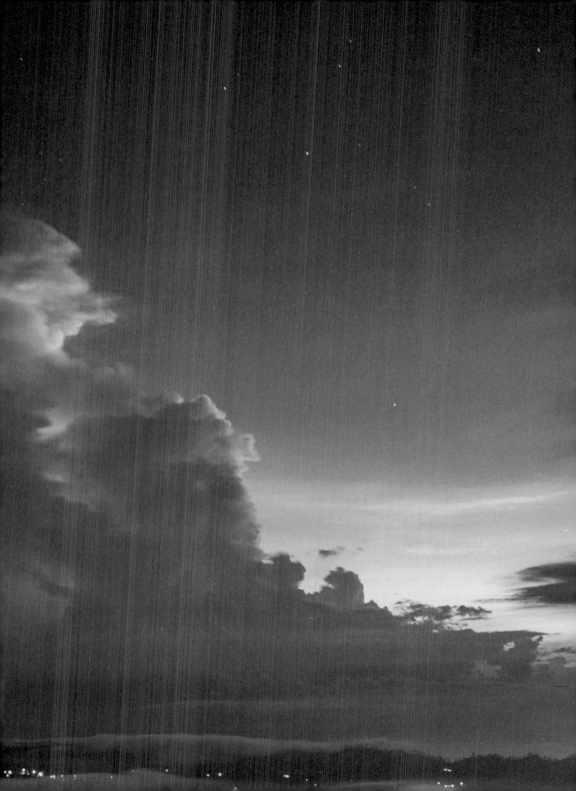

LUNAR CALENDAR

zone, please go to LunarAbundance.com/Free-Lunar-Planner

18	19	20	21	22	23	24	25	26	27	28	29	30	31

18	19	20	21	22	23	24	25	26	27	28	29	30	31

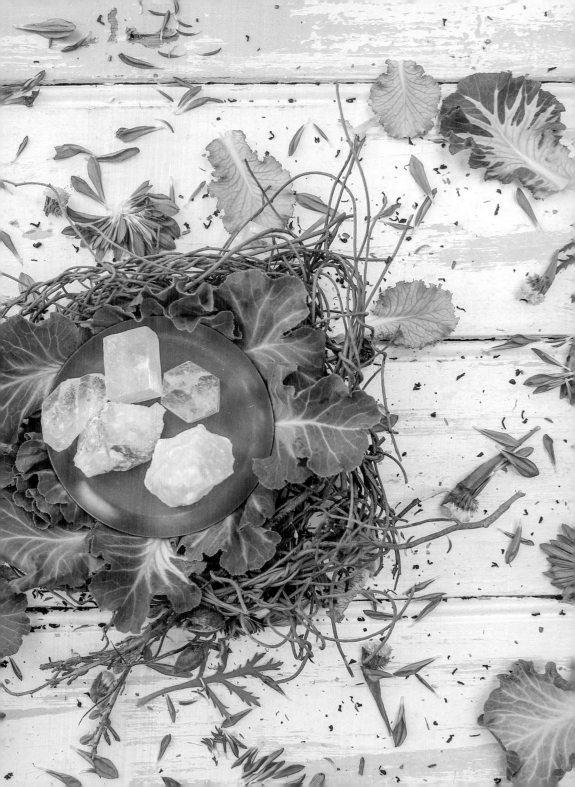

SUGGESTED READING

•

•

◖

◖

LUNAR CYCLES AND RESEARCH

Leonie A. Calver, Barrie J. Stokes, and Geoffrey K. Isbiste, "The Dark Side of the Moon," *Australian Medical Journal* 191, nos. 11–12 (2009): 692–694.

Cristy Gelling, "Full Moon May Mean Less Sleep: Slumber Waxes and Wanes with Lunar Cycles," *Society for Science and the Public* 184, no. 4 (2013): 15.

S. L. Gray and R. G. Harrison, "Diagnosing Eclipse-Induced Wind Change," *Proceedings of the Royal Society* 468 (2012): 1839–1850.

Sandra and David Mosley, *Zodiac Arts*, http://zodiacarts.com.

Ernest Naylor, *Moonstruck: How Lunar Cycles Affect Life* (Oxford University Press, 2015).

Richard D. Neal and Malcolm Colledge, "The Effect of the Full Moon on General Practice Consultation Rates," *Family Practice* 17, no. 6 (2000): 472–474.

Jack R. Pyle and Taylor Reese, *Raising with the Moon: The Complete Guide to Gardening and Living by the Signs of the Moon* (Parkway Publishers, 2003).

Dane Rudhyar, *The Lunation Cycle* (Llewellyn Publications, 1967).

Clive L. N. Ruggles, *Ancient Astronomy: An Encyclopedia of Cosmologies and Myth* (ABC-CLIO, 2005).

Michael Smithemail, Ilona Croy, and Kerstin Persson Waye, "Human Sleep and Cortical Reactivity Are Influenced by Lunar Phase," *Current Biology* 24, no. 12 (2014): R551–R552.

Rudolf Steiner, *Agriculture Course: The Birth of the Biodynamic Method*, translated by George Adams (Rudolf Steiner Press, 2014).

C. P. Thakur and Dilip Sharma, "Full Moon and Crime," *British Medical Journal* 289 no. 6460 (1984): 789–791.

David Whitehouse, *The Moon: A Biography* (Headline Book Publishing, 2001).

OTHER CYCLES

Edward Dewey and Edwin Dakin, *Cycles: The Science of Prediction* (Holt and Company, 1947).

George Haralambie, "The Global Crisis and Cyclical Theory," *Theoretical and Applied Economics* 11, no. 564 (2011): 79–88.

Rebecca Orleane, *The Return of the Feminine: Honoring the Cycles of Nature* (AuthorHouse, 2010).

BODY LOVE, SEXUALITY, AND SELF-ESTEEM

Saida Desilets, *The Emergence of the Sensual Woman—Awakening Our Erotic Innocence* (Jane Goddess Publishing, 2005).

Tracy Gaudet and Paula Spencer, *Consciously Female: How to Listen to Your Body and Your Soul for a Lifetime of Healthier Living* (Bantam, 2004).

Anita Johnston, *Eating in the Light of the Moon: How Women Can Transform Their Relationships with Food through Myths, Metaphors and Storytelling* (Gürze Books, 2000).

Azita Nahai, *Trauma to Dharma: Transform Your Pain Into Purpose* (AnR Books, 2018).

Christiane Northrup, *Women's Bodies, Women's Wisdom* (Piatkus Books, 1995).

SELECTED SOURCES ON SPIRITUALITY, JUNGIAN, AND DEPTH PSYCHOLOGY

Sera Beak, *Red Hot and Holy: A Heretic's Love Story* (Sounds True, 2013).

Tara Brach, *Radical Acceptance: Embracing Your Life with the Heart of a Buddha* (Bantam, 2004).

Tara Brach, *True Refuge: Finding Peace and Freedom in Your Own Awakened Heart* (Bantam, 2016).

Mariana Caplan, *Eyes Wide Open: Cultivating Discernment on the Spiritual Path* (Sounds True, 2009).

Pema Chödrön, *Living Beautifully: With Uncertainty and Change* (Shambhala Publications, 2012).

Thomas Cleary (ed. and trans.), *Immortal Sisters: Secret Teachings of Taoist Women* (North Atlantic Books, 1996).

Thomas Cleary (ed. and trans.), *Secret of the Golden Flower* (HarperCollins, 1993).

Thomas Cleary and Sartaz Aziz, *Twilight Goddess: Spiritual Feminism and Feminine Spirituality* (Shambhala Press, 2000).

Rose Mary Dougherty, *Discernment: A Path to Spiritual Awakening* (Paulist Press, 2009).

Judith Duerk, *Circle of Stones: Woman's Journey to Herself,* 10th anniversary ed. (New World Library, 2004).

Dr. Clarissa Pinkola Estés, *Women Who Run with the Wolves: Myths and Stories of the Wild Woman Archetype,* reprint ed. (Ballantine Books, 1996).

Kevin Farrow, *The Psychology of the Body* (AcuEnergetics Pty Ltd., 2007).

Kevin Farrow, *Meditation as Medicine* (AcuEnergetics Pty Ltd., 2010).

Kevin Farrow, *Enlighten: Practices for the Modern Mystic* (AcuEnergetics Pty Ltd., 2015).

Jentezen Franklin, *The Amazing Discernment of Women* (Nelson Books, 2006).

Dr. Carl Jung, *Collected Works* (Bollingen Foundation, 1993 [1952]).

Byron Katie, *Loving What Is: Four Questions That Can Change Your Life* (Three Rivers Press, 2003).

Byron Katie, *A Thousand Names for Joy: Living in Harmony with the Way Things Are* (Harmony, 2008).

Tami Lynn Kent, *Wild Feminine: Finding Power, Spirit and Joy in the Female Body* (Atria Books/Beyond Words, 2011).

Robert Augustus Masters, *Spiritual Bypassing: When Spirituality Disconnects Us from What Really Matters* (North Atlantic Books, 2010).

Maureen Murdock, *The Heroine's Journey* (Shambhala, 1990).

Rinpoche Dzogchen Ponlop, *Rebel Buddha: On the Road to Freedom* (Shambhala, 2011).

Barbara Schmidt, *The Practice: Simple Tools for Managing Stress, Finding Inner Peace, and Uncovering Happiness* (Health Communications, Inc., 2014).

Tosha Silver, *Outrageous Openness: Letting the Divine Take the Lead* (Atria Paperback, 2014).

Krista Tippett, *Becoming Wise: An Inquiry into the Mystery and Art of Living* (Penguin Press, 2016).

PERSONAL DEVELOPMENT, PRODUCTIVITY, AND LEADERSHIP

Dr. Brené Brown, *The Gifts of Imperfection: Let Go of Who You Think You're Supposed to Be and Embrace Who You Are* (Hazelden, 2010).

Dr. Brené Brown, *Rising Strong* (Vermilion Press, 2015).

P. R. Clance, and S. A. Imes, "The Impostor Phenomenon in High Achieving Women: Dynamics and Therapeutic Intervention," *Psychotherapy: Theory, Research, and Practice* 15, no. 3 (1978): 241–247.

Amy Cuddy, *Presence* (Little, Brown and Company, 2015).

Megan Dalla-Camina and Michelle McQuaid, *Lead Like a Woman: Your Essential Guide for True Confidence, Career Clarity, Vibrant Wellbeing and Leadership Success* (Lead Like a Woman Pty Ltd., 2016).

John Gerzema and Michael D'Antonio, *The Athena Doctrine: How Women (and the Men Who Think Like Them) Will Rule the Future* (Jossey-Bass, 2013).

Adam Grant, *Give and Take: A Revolutionary Approach to Success* (Penguin Press, 2014).

Greg McKeown, *Essentialism: The Disciplined Pursuit of Less* (Crown Business, 2014).

POWER OF REST, RELAXATION, AND BREATH

Ericsson K. Anders, Ralf T. Krampe, and Clemens Tesch-Römer, "The Role of Deliberate Practice in the Acquisition of Expert Performance," *Psychological Review* 100, no. 3 (1993): 363–406.

Benjamin Baird, Jonathan Smallwood, Michael D. Mrazek, Julia W. Y. Kam, Michael S. Franklin, and Jonathan W. Schooler, "Inspired by Distraction: Mind Wandering Facilitates Creative Incubation," *Psychological Science* 23, no. 10 (2010): 1117–1122.

Volker Busch, Walter Magerl, Uwe Kern, Joachim Haas, Göran Hajak, and Peter Eichhammer, "The Effect of Deep and Slow Breathing on Pain Perception, Autonomic Activity, and Mood Processing—An Experimental Study," *The American Academy of Pain Medicine* 13, no. 2 (2011): 215–228.

Ap Dijksterhuis, Maarten W. Bos, Loran F. Nordgren, and Rick B. van Baaren, "On Making the Right Choice: The Deliberation-without-Attention Effect," *Science* 311, no. 5763 (2006): 1005–1007.

Mary Helen Immordino-Yang, Joanna A. Christodoulou, and Vanessa Singh, "Rest Is Not Idleness: Implications of the Brain's Default Mode for Human Development and Education," *Perspectives on Psychological Science* 7, no. 4 (2012): 352–364.

Ravinder Jerath and Vernon A. Barnes, "Augmentation of Mind-Body Therapy and Role of Deep Slow Breathing," *Journal of Complementary and Integrative Medicine* 13, no. 2 (2011): 566–571.

Ravinder Jerath, Vernon A. Barnes, Molly W. Crawford, and Kyler Harden, "Self-Regulation of Breathing as a Primary Treatment for Anxiety," *Applied Psychophysiology and Biofeedback* 40 (2015): 107–111.

Ravinder Jerath, J. W. Edry, Vernon A. Barnes, and Vandna Jerath, "Physiology of Long Pranayamic Breathing: Neural Respiratory Elements May Provide a Mechanism That Explains How Slow Deep Breathing Shifts the Autonomic Nervous System," *Medical Hypotheses* 67, no. 3 (2006): 566–571.

FEELING AND EXPRESSING EMOTIONS

Benjamin P. Chapman, Kevin Fiscella, Ichiro Kawachi, Paul Duberstein, and Peter Muennig, "Emotion Suppression and Mortality Risk Over a 12-Year Follow-Up," *Journal of Psychosomatic Research* 75, no. 4 (2013): 381–385.

Gordon L. Flett, Paul L. Hewitt and Marnin J. Heisel, "The Destructiveness of Perfectionism Revisited: Implications for the Assessment of Suicide Risk and the Prevention of Suicide," *Review of General Psychology* 18, no. 3 (2014): 156–172.

X. D. Martin and M. C. Brennan, "Serotonin in Human Tears," *European Journal of Ophthalmology* 4, no. 3 (1994): 159–165.

Judith Orloff, *Emotional Freedom: Liberate Yourself from Negative Emotions and Transform Your Life* (Harmony, 2010).

James W. Pennebaker, *Opening Up: The Healing Power of Expressing Emotions*, 2nd ed. (The Guilford Press, 1990).

Michael Philp, Sarah Egan, and Robert Kane, "Perfectionism, Over Commitment to Work, and Burnout in Employees Seeking Workplace Counselling," *Australian Journal of Psychology* 64 (2012): 68–74.

Julie Sheldon, *The Blessing of Tears* (Hymns Ancient and Modern Ltd., 2004).

Philip M. Ullirch and Susan K. Lutgendorf, "Journalling About Stressful Events: Effects of Cognitive Processing and Emotional Expression," *Annals of Behavioural Medicine* 24, no. 3 (2002): 244–250.

Els van der Helm, Ninad Gujar, and Matthew P. Walker, "Sleep Deprivation Impairs the Accurate Recognition of Human Emotions," *Sleep* 33, no. 3 (2010): 335–342.

Ad Vingerhoets, *Why Only Humans Weep: Unravelling the Mysteries of Tears* (Oxford University Press, 2013).

PSYCHOLOGY AND NEUROPSYCHOLOGY

Norman Doidge, *The Brain that Changes Itself* (Penguin Books, 2008).

James Doty, *Into the Magic Shop*, 2nd ed. (Avery, 2016).

Williams James, *The Principles of Psychology* (Holt, 1890).

Thomas Pink, *The Psychology of Freedom* (Cambridge University Press, 1996).

American Psychological Association, "Suppressing the 'White Bears,'" https://www.apa.org/monitor/2011/10/unwanted-thoughts.

STAY CONNECTED

LUNAR ABUNDANCE WEBSITE

Visit my website, LunarAbundance.com, for free graphics and audio resources about this lunar practice, download your free lunar planner with the dates of all eight Moon phases for the year, and sign up for free e-letters that will remind you of the time and date of each upcoming New and Full Moon. You will also find journaling resources to help you develop your practice.

LUNAR ABUNDANCE SALON

Join the Lunar Abundance Salon, an online program where we delve much more deeply into this practice by following the Moon for a full solar year, working with several specific intention themes and aspects of abundance.

SOCIAL MEDIA

Come and say hi to me on social media, and share your experiences (I love to hear from you!):

Instagram @ezziespencer

Facebook @lunarabundance

ACKNOWLEDGMENTS

With thanks to my meticulous editor Cindy Sipala at Running Press and my wonderful agent Meg Thompson for encouraging me to write this very practical follow-up to the original *Lunar Abundance* book. Thank you to all my teachers, to Emma-Kate Codrington for the beautiful Lunar Abundance photos, and the spectacular designer Sarah Gleeson for helping me to create the contemplative Moon graphics. Much gratitude to the Assemblage for providing such a nurturing home base for my writing and teaching in New York City.

Most of all, I have deep appreciation for the tens of thousands of readers who follow the Lunar Abundance practice, email me, follow me on Instagram, and come to my regular live events. This practice has only become what it is because YOU breathe life into it. Thank you!

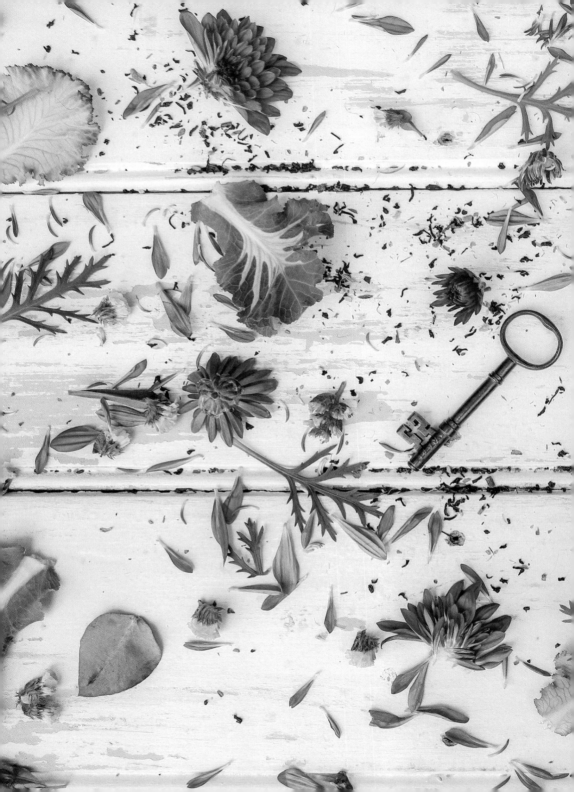

ABOUT THE AUTHOR

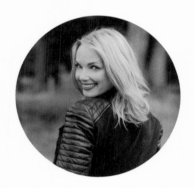

EZZIE SPENCER, PhD is the author of *Lunar Abundance* (2018). Through one-on-one coaching and as the creator of Lunar Abundance—a lunar-inspired, holistic self-care practice—Ezzie helps people around the world cultivate self-worth, creativity, and confidence. Originally from Australia, she lives in Brooklyn, New York.

Author Photo © In Her Image Photography

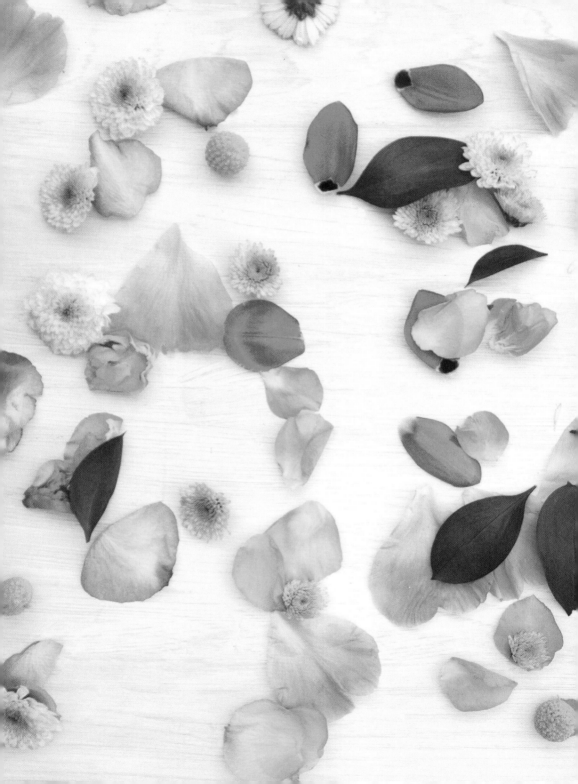